www.harcourt-international.com

Bringing you products from all Harcourt Health Sciences companies including Bailli… …e, Mosby and W.B. Saunders

- **Browse** for latest info… …s and electronic products
- **Search** for information on over 20 000 published titles with full product information including tables of contents and sample chapters
- **Keep up to date** with our extensive publishing programme in your field by registering with eAlert or requesting postal updates
- **Secure online ordering** with prompt delivery, as well as full contact details to order by phone, fax or post
- **News** of special features and promotions

If you are based in the following countries, please visit the country-specific site to receive full details of product availability and local ordering information

USA: www.harcourthealth.com

Canada: www.harcourtcanada.com

Australia: www.harcourt.com

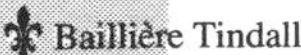

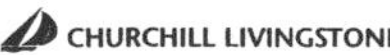

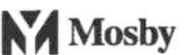

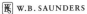

For Churchill Livingstone

Senior Commissioning Editor: Sarena Wolfaard
Project Development Manager: Dinah Thom
Designer: George Ajayi

Using Maths in Health Sciences

Chris Gunn MA TDCR
CG Training, Retford, Nottinghamshire, UK

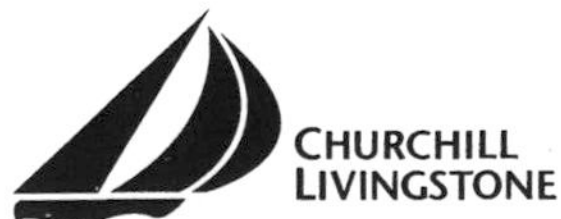

EDINBURGH LONDON NEW YORK PHILADELPHIA
ST LOUIS SYDNEY TORONTO 2001

CHURCHILL LIVINGSTONE
An imprint of Harcourt Publishers Limited

First published 2001
Transferred to Digital Printing 2005

ISBN 0 443 07074 1

British Library Cataloguing in Publication Data
A catalogue record for this book is available from the British Library

Library of Congress Cataloging in Publication Data
A catalog record for this book is available from the Library of Congress

The Publisher's policy is to use paper manufactured from sustainable forests

Printed and bound by Antony Rowe Ltd, Eastbourne

Contents

Preface

In spite of the title, this is not a maths book. It was written with the assumption that users would have been taught how to do the maths covered in the book. Unfortunately, when people are not doing the same calculations day after day there is a tendency to forget basic formulae and the order of working. This publication therefore aims to provide the basic *aide-mémoire* for students and staff who have to do calculations but need a reminder of the technique used.

The book is divided into three sections. The first covers statistics, as there is an increasing demand for this type of work. There is a glossary of statistical terms and a table indicating which statistical test to select. The second section covers worked, practical examples, and the final part includes some of the basic maths required to do the worked examples.

As the use of computers and calculators is increasing, examples of spreadsheets, the use of Excel and the use of calculators have been briefly included. Throughout the book numbers in boxes refer to the keys to be pressed when using a calculator, as it was felt that this was the easiest way to give the information.

I would like to thank the following people who have assisted with this publication: Don Gunn for checking the calculations and assisting with the compilation of the statistical tables; John Buckley, at the Department of Exercise and Sports Science, Manchester Metropolitan University, for providing examples of sports questions; Kevin Kelly and Graham Hutchesson for commenting on the statistical section of the book.

Retford, Nottinghamshire 2000 Chris Gunn

SECTION ONE
Basic statistics

3.78

0.378

0.0378

1. Graphs

A graph shows the link between two groups of data

AXES

Two lines at right angles to each other
Horizontal line is called the x axis
NB: x goes **across**
Vertical line is called the y axis
Where the axes meet is usually 0

SCALES

A sequence of numbers
Either increasing or decreasing in order
Log numbers can be used to enable a very large or very small range of numbers to be fitted on to the graph

Logarithms p. 162

CARTESIAN CO-ORDINATES

Position of the point (P) on a graph
The plot is the point where the value of x meets the value of y
NB: the value of x is always given first

Example

If $x = 2$ and $y = 3$, plot P

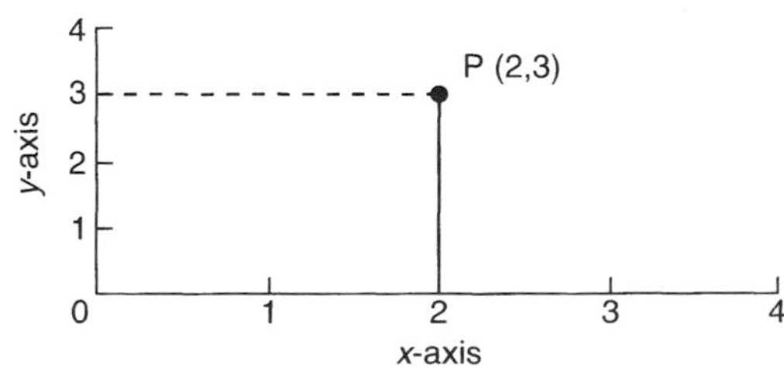

DRAWING A GRAPH

PREPARATION

1 Collect the data (numbers being used)

2 Decide the scale, for example:

x = years, y = number of patients (in thousands)
or x = hours, y = number of consultations

Example

Data

x = age in years	y = number of patients
5	14
6	36
7	12
8	16
9	40
10	3

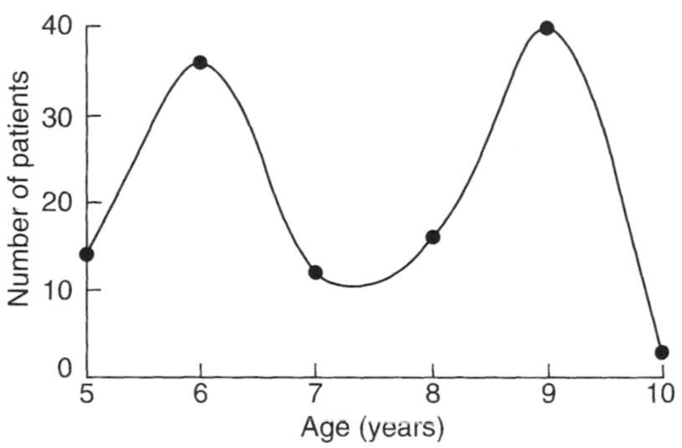

PLOTTING GRAPHS USING EXCEL

TO CREATE A GRAPH

- Open Excel
- In A1 type the title of the x axis
- In B1, C1, D1, etc. type the data for the x axis
- In A2 type the title for the y axis
- In B2, C2, D2, etc. type the data for the y axis
- Click Insert and select Chart
- Select the type of graph required, click Next
- Click on data range and then left-click on boxes B1, B2, C1, C2, D1, D2, etc., click Next
- Add the chart title in the box provided
- Name the x axis
- Give the range of values for the y axis, and click Next
- To save on the same sheet as the data, save object in Sheet 1, click Finish

TO CHANGE THE GRAPH

- Click on the appropriate area of the graph, e.g. to make a histogram create a bar chart and then click on an individual bar to widen it

TO COPY TO A WORD DOCUMENT

- Open the word document and minimise the screen by clicking on [_] in the top right-hand corner

- Open Excel and the page with the saved graph. **NB**: if you cannot see the minimised Word document click View, click Full screen (this will minimise the size of the screen)
- Right-click on the graph and, on the drop-down window, left-click on Copy (a pulsating dotted line appears round the graph)
- Click on the minimised Word document to restore the window
- Select where you wish the graph to appear, light-click on the document, click on Paste

2. The range

The range is found by taking the highest and lowest numbers in a series

Example

2 4 6 8 10 = 2 to 10

and by taking the lowest from the highest

Therefore the range = 10 − 2 = 8

USEFUL

- When all the numbers in the series cluster together

NOT USEFUL

- If the values are widely spread
- If the values are unevenly distributed

3. Probability

Probability (P) is the likelihood of something happening
Probability can be described as a ratio, a percentage or a decimal

Example
Take the word PROBABILITY, which has 11 letters.
If the letters were placed in a bag the:

- probability of a letter A being pulled out would be:

  $\frac{1}{11}$ or 9% or 0.09

- probability of a vowel (o, a, i, i) being pulled out would be:

  $\frac{4}{11}$ or 36% or 0.36

- probability of a consonant (p, r, b, b, l, t, y) being pulled out would be:

  $\frac{7}{11}$ or 63% or 0.63

4. Ranking sets of scores

Ranking is the method of organising data

Example

Rank: 9 11 3 5 9 7 10 9 5 11 3

1 Starting with the smallest, write the scores in order of size
3 3 5 5 7 9 9 9 10 11 11

2 Number from the left
3 3 5 5 7 9 9 9 10 11 11
1 2 3 4 5 6 7 8 9 10 11

3 If there are several numbers the same (i.e. tied) select the number between (i.e. add together the ranks of the tied numbers and divide by the number of numbers that were added together)
3 3 5 5 7 9 9 9 10 11 11
1.5 1.5 3.5 3.5 5 7 7 7 9 10.5 10.5

4 Write in a vertical column

Score	Rank
3	**1.5**
3	**1.5**
5	**3.5**
5	**3.5**
7	**5**
9	**7**
9	**7**
9	**7**
10	**9**
11	**10.5**
11	**10.5**

5. Frequency distribution

Frequency is when some results occur more than once
The frequency distribution is the number of times each result appears in a table
It is a way of organising data to make the results clearer

Example

1 Starting with the smallest, write the scores in order of size

1 2 2 2 3 3 3 3 4 4 5 6

2 Count the number of times each score occurs

1 2 2 2 3 3 3 3 4 4 5 6
1 3 3 3 4 4 4 4 2 2 1 1

3 Write in list or table form

Score	Frequency
1	1
2	3
2	3
2	3
3	4
3	4
3	4
3	4
4	2
4	2
5	1
6	1

6. The mean ($\bar{x}$)

TO CALCULATE

Add the scores together and divide by the number of scores you add up, this gives the mean (or average; $\bar{x}$)

Example

$$23 + 25 + 24 + 23 + 20 = 115$$
$$115 \div 5 = 23$$

USEFUL

- If the scores cluster round one number
- Can be calculated exactly
- Can be used in later work

NOT USEFUL

- If the original scores are widely spread
- If the original scores are unevenly distributed
- If the original scores cluster at the extremes
- If the answer is not a whole number, e.g. 2.35 children

Formula

$$\bar{x} = \frac{\sum x}{N}$$

$\sum$ = sigma = sum of
x = the individual score
N = the total number of scores

7. The median

TO CALCULATE

Arrange the numbers in the order of size and select the number that falls in the middle

Example

2 4 6 8 10 12 14

The median = 8

For an even number of numbers, add the two central numbers together and divide by 2

Example

2 4 6 8 10 12 14 16

$8 + 10 = 18$

$18 \div 2 = 9$

The median = 9

USEFUL

- For small groups of numbers
- If one of the extreme values changes in value (as this will not affect the result)
- If some numbers are clearly out of line with the others (outliers) – the median should be the description of choice
- If the scores have an uneven pattern
- To represent scores that have too high or too low values (e.g. if a test was too easy or too difficult for the participants)

NOT USEFUL

- For very large groups of numbers (time consuming)
- Unreliable if one of the central values changes
- If one of the extreme values disappears (as this will change the median)

8. The mode

TO CALCULATE

Find the number that occurs most often in a series

Frequency distribution p. 10

Example

2 2 3 3 3 4 4 4 4 4

As the number 4 occurs five times, the mode = 4

If more groups of numbers occur

Example

2 3 4 4 4 5 6 6 6

In the above example there are two modes – 4 and 6

Therefore the set is described as being bimodal.

USEFUL

- Used to indicate the most 'usual' or typical score
- Useful if the number are not evenly spread, e.g.
  1 2 5 7 7 8 8 8 9
  the mode = 8

NOT USEFUL

- It is possible for the scores to have a number of modes – therefore the more modes the less useful the term
- The mode can be very unstable as adding a single number can change the mode, e.g.
  2 2 3 4 5
  the mode = 2
  But if another score of 5 is added it becomes bimodal

9. Measures of central tendency

These can be the:

- mean
- median
- mode

The measure selected should be the one that best describes the information (statistics) being represented

NB: Selecting the incorrect measure can mislead the reader

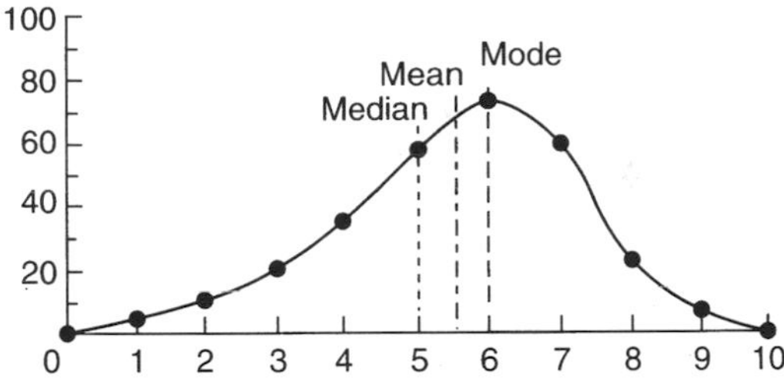

10. Normal distribution (*Z*)

The pattern in which most data falls
The mean, median and mode are close together
There are very few, very low or very high scores
The curve is described as being 'bell shaped'

PROPERTIES

- The mean, median and mode lie at the central point
- By calculating the standard deviation (SD) for the curve it is possible to plot the spread of data above and below the mean
- 1 SD either side of the mean will cover about 68% of the scores
- 2 SD either side of the mean will cover about 95% of the scores
- 3 SD either side of the mean will cover about 99% of the scores
- 4 SD either side of the mean will cover about 99.9% of the scores

Formula

$$Z = \frac{x - \bar{x}}{\text{SD}}$$

x = score
$\bar{x}$ = mean
SD = standard deviation

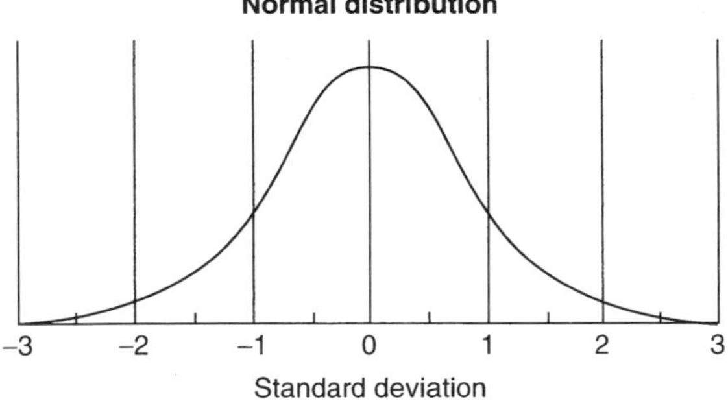

NORMAL DISTRIBUTION TABLE

The table is for one-tailed tests
For two-tailed tests, double the probabilities

Z	.00	.01	.02	.03	.04	.05	.06	.07	.08	.09
0.0	.5000	.4960	.4920	.4880	.4840	.4801	.4761	.4721	.4681	.4641
0.1	.4602	.4562	.4522	.4483	.4443	.4404	.4364	.4325	.4286	.4247
0.2	.4207	.4168	.4129	.4090	.4052	.4013	.3974	.3936	.3897	.3859
0.3	.3821	.3783	.3745	.3707	.3669	.3632	.3594	.3557	.3520	.3483
0.4	.3446	.3409	.3372	.3336	.3300	.3264	.3228	.3192	.3156	.3121
0.5	.3085	.3050	.3015	.2981	.2946	.2912	.2877	.2843	.2810	.2776
0.6	.2743	.2709	.2676	.2643	.2611	.2578	.2546	.2514	.2483	.2451
0.7	.2420	.2389	.2358	.2327	.2296	.2266	.2236	.2206	.2177	.2148
0.8	.2119	.2090	.2061	.2033	.2005	.1977	.1949	.1922	.1894	.1867
0.9	.1814	.1841	.1788	.1762	.1736	.1711	.1685	.1660	.1635	.1611
1.0	.1587	.1562	.1539	.1515	.1492	.1469	.1446	.1423	.1401	.1379
1.1	.1357	.1335	.1314	.1292	.1271	.1251	.1230	.1210	.1190	.1170
1.2	.1151	.1131	.1112	.1093	.1075	.1056	.1038	.1020	.1003	.0985
1.3	.0968	.0951	.0934	.0918	.0901	.0885	.0869	.0853	.0838	.0823
1.4	.0808	.0793	.0778	.0764	.0749	.0735	.0721	.0708	.0694	.0681
1.5	.0668	.0655	.0643	.0630	.0618	.0606	.0594	.0582	.0571	.0559
1.6	.0548	.0537	.0526	.0516	.0505	.0495	.0485	.0475	.0465	.0455
1.7	.0446	.0436	.0427	.0418	.0409	.0401	.0392	.0384	.0375	.0367
1.8	.0359	.0351	.0344	.0366	.0329	.0322	.0314	.0307	.0301	.0294
1.9	.0287	.0281	.0274	.0268	.0262	.0256	.0250	.0244	.0239	.0233
2.0	.0228	.0222	.0217	.0212	.0207	.0202	.0197	.0192	.0188	.0183
2.1	.0179	.0174	.0170	.0166	.0162	.0158	.0154	.0150	.0146	.0143
2.2	.0139	.0136	.0132	.0129	.0125	.0122	.0119	.0116	.0113	.0110
2.3	.0107	.0104	.0102	.0099	.0096	.0094	.0091	.0089	.0087	.0084
2.4	.0082	.0080	.0078	.0075	.0073	.0071	.0069	.0068	.0066	.0064
2.5	.0062	.0060	.0059	.0057	.0055	.0054	.0052	.0051	.0049	.0048
2.6	.0047	.0045	.0044	.0043	.0041	.0040	.0039	.0038	.0037	.0036
2.7	.0035	.0034	.0033	.0032	.0031	.0030	.0029	.0028	.0027	.0026
2.8	.0026	.0025	.0024	.0023	.0023	.0022	.0021	.0021	.0020	.0019
2.9	.0019	.0018	.0018	.0017	.0016	.0016	.0015	.0015	.0014	.0014
3.0	.0013	.0013	.0013	.0012	.0012	.0012	.0011	.0011	.0010	.0010

Glossary p. 67–68

11. Standard deviation

USE

To calculate the standard deviation of a set of data

REQUIRE

Data of interval status *Statistical glossary p. 66*

METHOD

1 Count the number of scores (N)

2 Find the mean of the scores ($\bar{x}$) *The mean p. 11*

3 Take the mean from each individual score and square the result

4 Add together the calculated squares

5 Divide the sum of the squares by $N - 1$ to give the variance

6 Square root the variance to give the standard deviation (SD)

Formula

$$\sqrt{\left(\frac{\sum(x - \bar{x})^2}{N - 1}\right)}$$

$\sum$ = sum
x = individual scores
$\bar{x}$ = mean of the scores
N = number of scores

Example

Data = 10, 15, 18, 19, 23

1 Count the number of scores: $N = 5$

2 Find the mean of the scores, $\bar{x}$:

$$\frac{10 + 15 + 18 + 19 + 23}{5} = 17$$

3 Take the mean from each individual score and square the result

$10 - 17 = -7$ squared $= 49$

$15 - 17 = -2$ squared $= 4$

$18 - 17 = 1$ squared $= 1$

$19 - 17 = 2$ squared $= 4$

$23 - 17 = 6$ squared $= 36$

4 Add the calculated squares together

$49 + 4 + 1 + 4 + 36 = 94$

5 Divide the sum of the squares by $N - 1$

$94 \div (5 - 1) =$ variance $= 23.5$

6 Square root the variance

$\sqrt{23.5} = 4.85$

Standard deviation (SD) = 4.85

STANDARD DEVIATION – USING A SPREADSHEET

From the previous example enter:

	A	B	C	D
1	10	= (A1 – D1)^2		= A6/5
2	15	= (A2 – D1)^2		= B6/4
3	18	= (A3 – D1)^2		= SQRT (D2)
4	19	= (A4 – D1)^2		
5	23	= (A5 – D1)^2		
6	= SUM (A1:A5)	= SUM (B1:B5)		

See the Excel section of the Statistical glossary for a definition of the terms used (p. 69).

Step 1 = A6 **Step 4** = B6

Step 2 = D1 **Step 5** = D2

Step 3 = B1 to B5 **Step 6** = D3

The result in a spreadsheet is:

	A	B	C	D
1	10	49		17
2	15	4		23.5
3	18	1		4.85
4	19	4		
5	23	36		
	85	94		

12. Pie charts

Display information as a proportion of the whole
Useful when wishing to visually compare individual areas
Ideally no more than six sections should be used, with a maximum of eight, or the results will be difficult to read

Example

A survey of waiting times for 100 patients

Waiting time (in minutes)	Number of patients
0–10	3
11–20	27
21–30	45
31–40	15
41–50	6
Over 51	4

There are 360° in a circle. To find how many degrees one person represents, divide 360 by the total number of patients:

360 **÷** **100** **=** **3.6**

To find the angle for each group, multiply the angle for one person by the number of people in the group:

3.6 **×** **3** **=** **11°**

(The answer is to the nearest degree)

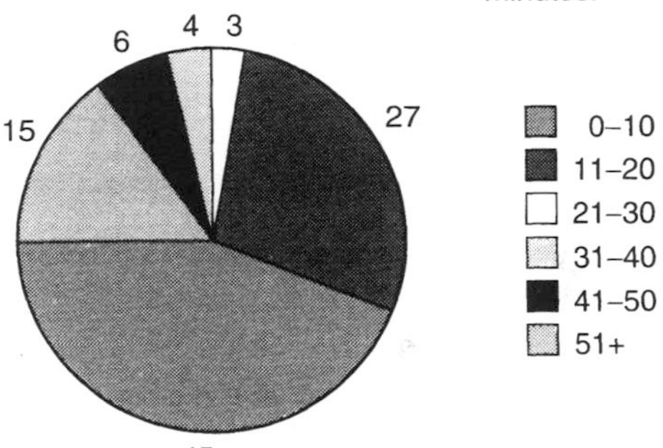
Pie chart
Numbers of patients waiting:
Waiting time in minutes:
6
4
3
27
15
45
0–10
11–20
21–30
31–40
41–50
51+

13. Bar charts

Bar charts can be drawn vertically or horizontally
The height (or length) of the bar gives the number of items
They show comparisons between various items, e.g. patients, conditions, etc.
It is difficult to determine the total of all items

Example

Cigarette smoking related to socioeconomic group

Group	Number of cigarettes smoked per 1000 population
Professional	25
Managerial	40
Skilled manual	50
Semi-skilled	53
Unskilled	60

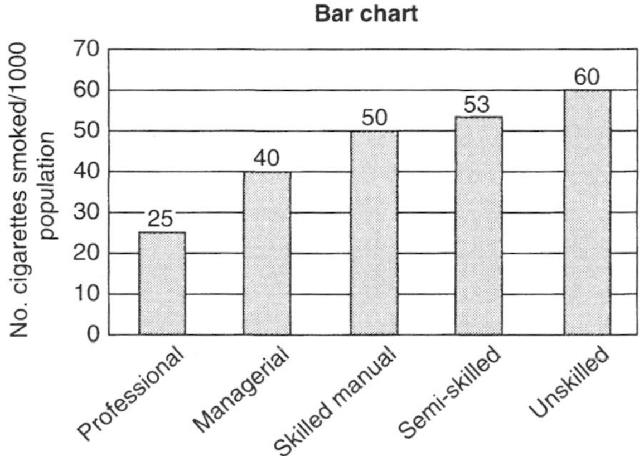

14. Histograms

A graph in which frequency distribution is shown by rectangles (similar to a bar chart)
The rectangles are placed together as they are related to each other
Useful for showing the frequency of a set of results
Remember, a graph shows a link between two groups of numbers

Example

Weight in kg	40–50	51–55	56–60	61–65
Number of women	2	4	19	27

Weight in kg	66–70	71–75	76–80	81–85
Number of women	60	45	26	18

Weight in kg	86–90	91–95		
Number of women	5	1		

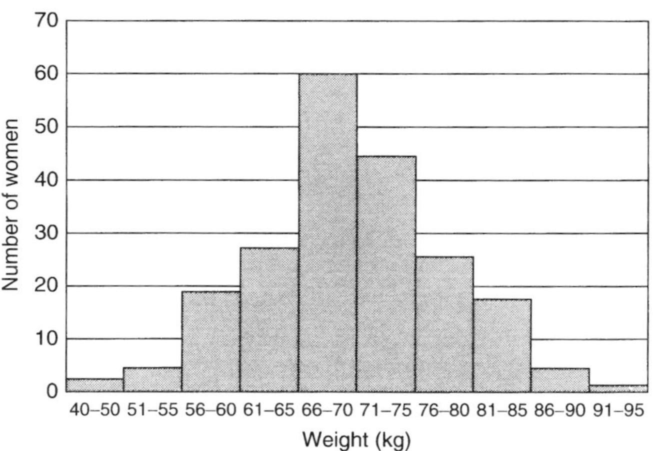
70
60
50
40
30
20
10
0
Number of women
40–50 51–55 56–60 61–65 66–70 71–75 76–80 81–85 86–90 91–95
Weight (kg)

15. Scattergrams

A method of visually representing two variables
For a perfect correlation the points will lie in approximately a straight line
The less perfect the correlation the more the plots will resemble an oval
If the plots represent an oval there is no correlation

Example

x axis	0	3	4	4	5	5	5	6	7	8	8	9	10
y axis	0	7	4	5	5	7	9	2	9	4	6	8	3

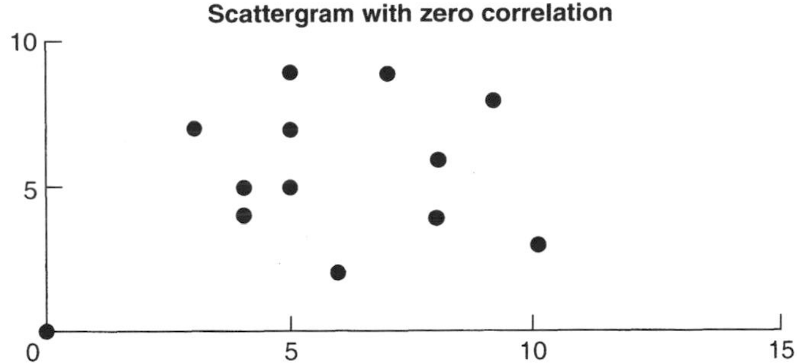

16. Correlation

Correlation means 'associated with'
Correlation coefficients show the degree of association between two variables *Glossary p. 66*
There are two types of correlation; positive and negative
Correlation is a measure of cause and effect

POSITIVE CORRELATION

- Occurs when data is linked
- More of one will result in more of the other
- Less of one will result in less of the other

Example

The more exercise taken the greater the weight loss

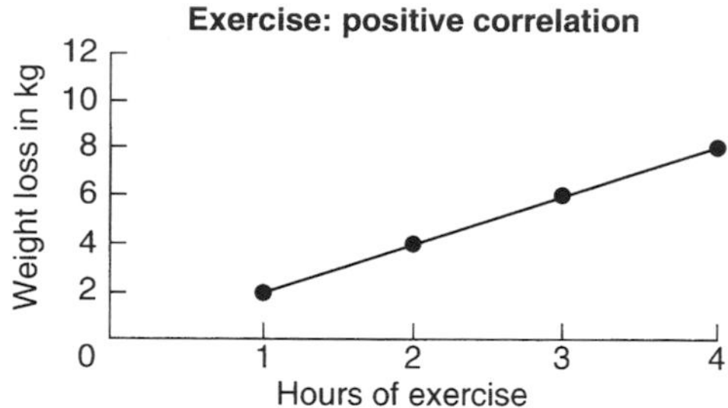

NEGATIVE CORRELATION

- Occurs when data is linked
- An increase in one item will result in a decrease in the other
- A decrease in one item will result in an increase in the other

Example

The more items bought the less money available. The fewer items bought the more money available

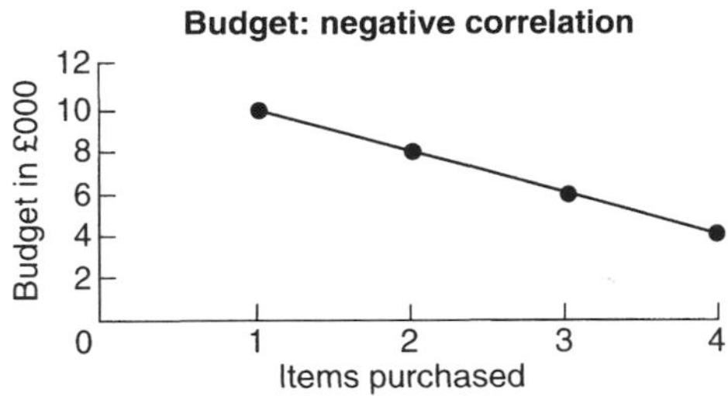

17. Which statistical test?

Data can be:

Nominal an allocated number, a method of classification

Ordinal indicating an order or rank in a sequence

Interval the numbers are ordinal and the steps between each number are of equal size

Related the data is matched – each individual sample has a matched sample with one or more than one variable in common

Unrelated the whole group is roughly matched but the individual samples are not

Parametric the scores are from a normal population and when plotted would give a normal distribution curve. The data is interval. The test is therefore powerful

Non-parametric no assumptions are made about the distribution. The data is ordinal. The tests are less powerful

Actual scores each score has a real value

RELATED DATA

	Nominal	Ordinal	Interval
Parametric			Related *t*-test
Non-parametric	Sign test	Wilcoxon	

UNRELATED DATA

	Nominal	Ordinal	Interval
Parametric			Unrelated *t*-test
Non-parametric	Chi-square test	Mann–Whitney *U* test	

18. Sign test

USE

When comparing two sets of results, i.e. paired results

REQUIRE

Paired data

Table of critical values of S

Sign test table p. 34

Normal distribution table

Normal distribution table p. 18

RESULTS

S must be equal to or less than the reading on the tables to be significant

METHOD

1 For each pair, take value b from value a. If the answers are positive mark +, if negative mark – (ignore any 0s)
2 To find S, count the number of times the least common sign appears
3 To calculate N, count the number of signs (excluding any signs with a difference of 0)
4 Decide if the test is one-tailed or two-tailed

Statistical glossary pp. 67–68

5 Using the table read off at the level N.
6 For one-tailed tests, if S is equal to or greater than the stated number given in the table the result is not significant
7 For two-tailed tests, the significance levels should be multiplied by 2

Example

Subject	Rating a	Rating b	Subject	Rating a	Rating b
1	6	2	**6**	9	2
2	4	9	**7**	7	4
3	7	3	**8**	3	9
4	4	8	**9**	6	4
5	6	1	**10**	8	4

1 Take rating b from rating a

$6 - 2 = +4,\ 4 - 9 = -5,\ 7 - 3 = +4,\ 4 - 8 = -4,$
$6 - 1 = +5,\ 9 - 2 = +7,\ 7 - 4 = +3,\ 3 - 9 = -6,$
$6 - 4 = +2,\ 8 - 4 = +4$

2 Number of positive results = 7, number of negative results =3

Therefore $S = 3$

3 Count the total number of signs (excluding any pairs with the difference of 0)

$N = 10$

4 Using the table at level $N = 10$. As S is greater than the numbers given, the result is not significant

SIGN TEST TABLE

Level of significance for one-tailed tests
For two-tailed test, multiply significance level (degrees of freedom; *df*) by 2

N \ *df*	0.10	0.05	0.02	0.01	0.001
5	0	–	–	–	–
6	0	0	–	–	–
7	0	0	0	–	–
8	1	0	0	0	–
9	1	1	0	0	0
10	1	1	0	0	0
11	2	1	1	0	0
12	2	2	1	1	0
13	3	2	1	1	0
14	3	2	2	1	0
15	3	3	2	2	1
16	4	3	2	2	1
17	4	4	3	2	1
18	5	4	3	3	1
19	5	4	4	3	2
20	5	5	4	3	2

SIGN TEST WHEN *N* IS LARGER THAN 25

Formula

$$Z = \frac{0.5 \times N - T - 0.5}{0.5 \times \sqrt{N}}$$

Z = value of the standard deviation
N = the number of pairs
T = the number of times the least common sign appears

Example

If you have a total of 70 pairs and 55 are ranked positive and 10 are ranked negative, calculate the significance

$N = 70$

$T = 10$

Therefore

$$Z = \frac{0.5 \times 70 - 10 - 0.5}{0.5 \times \sqrt{70}}$$
$$= \frac{24.5}{4.1833}$$
$$Z = 5.8566$$

Using the normal distribution table on page 18,
0.05 is at the level of 1.64
As the value of Z is greater than 1.64, the results would be significant at the 5% level (i.e. 0.05)

19. Wilcoxon test

USE

When comparing two sets of results, i.e. paired results

REQUIRE

Paired data (matched data)

Table of critical values of *T* for the Wilcoxon matched pairs signed rank test *Wilcoxon test table p. 38*

Normal distribution table *Normal distribution table p. 18*

RESULTS

T must be equal to or less than the reading on the tables to be significant

METHOD

1 For each pair, take the values of b from the values of a

2 Rank the answers (ignore any 0s) *Ranking p. 9*

3 Add the positive ranks together

4 Add the negative ranks together

5 Whichever is the smallest total in steps **3** and **4** gives the test statistic *T*

6 To calculate *N*, count the number of pairs (excluding any pairs with a difference of 0)

7 Using the table, read off at the level *N* and find the number that is equal to or larger than *T*

8 For one-tailed tests, if *T* is equal to or less than the stated number it is significant

9 For two-tailed tests, the significance levels should be multiplied by 2

Example

Subject	Rating a	Rating b	Subject	Rating a	Rating b
1	6	2	6	9	2
2	4	9	7	7	4
3	7	3	8	3	9
4	4	8	9	6	4
5	6	1	10	8	4

1 Take rating b from rating a

$6 - 2 = 4,\ 4 - 9 = -5,\ 7 - 3 = 4,\ 4 - 8 = -4,$
$6 - 1 = 5,\ 9 - 2 = 7,\ 7 - 4 = 3,\ 3 - 9 = -6,$
$6 - 4 = 2,\ 8 - 4 = 4$

2 Rank answers (ignore any 0s and −signs)

Difference	2	3	4	4	4	−4	5	−5	−6	7
Rank	1	2	4.5	4.5	4.5	4.5	7.5	7.5	9	10

3 Add positive ranks $= 1 + 2 + 4.5 + 4.5 + 4.5 + 7.5 + 10 = 34$

4 Add negative ranks $= 4.5 + 7.5 + 9 = 21$

5 The smallest total in steps **3** and **4** gives the test statistic T. Therefore $T = 21$

6 Count the number of pairs (excluding any pairs with the difference of 0), $N = 10$

7 Using the Wilcoxon test table at level $N = 10$ none of the values are equal to or just larger than the value of T, therefore there is no significant difference between the two sets of results

WILCOXON TEST TABLE

Level of significance for two-tailed tests For one-tailed test divide significance level by 2				
N	**0.10**	**0.05**	**0.02**	**0.01**
5	0.5	–	–	–
6	2	0.5	–	–
7	3.5	2	0	–
8	5.5	3.5	1.5	0
9	7	5.5	3	1.5
10	10.5	8	5	3
11	13.5	11	7	5
12	17	13.5	9.5	7
13	21	17	12.5	9.5
14	25.5	21	15.5	12.5
15	30	25	19.5	15.5
16	35.5	29.5	23.5	19.5
17	41	34.5	27.5	23
18	47	40	32.5	27.5
19	53.5	46	37.5	32
20	60	52	43	37.5
21	67.5	58.5	49	42.5
22	75	66	55.5	48.5
23	83	73	62	54.5
24	91.5	81	69	61

WILCOXON TEST WHEN *N* IS LARGER THAN 25

Formula

$$Z = \frac{T - \frac{N(N+1)}{4}}{\sqrt{\frac{N(N+1)(2N+1)}{24}}}$$

Z = Value of the standard deviation
N = the number of pairs (ignoring those with a difference of 0)
T = sum of the ranks with the less frequent sign

Example

If you have a total of 70 pairs and the sum of the ranks with the less frequent sign = 150, calculate the significance

$$N = 70$$

$$T = 150$$

$$Z = \frac{150 - \frac{70(70+1)}{4}}{\sqrt{\frac{70(70+1)(2\times 70+1)}{24}}}$$

$$= \frac{150 - 1242.5}{\sqrt{29198.75}}$$

$$= \frac{-1192.5}{170.876}$$

$$Z = -6.97$$

Using the normal distribution table on page 18,
0.05 is at the level of 1.64

As the value of Z is greater than 1.64 the results would be significant at the 5% level (i.e. 0.05)

NB: Z is usually negative, but this does not affect the interpretation

20. Simple chi-square test (χ^2)

USE

To compare groups where their observed behaviour has been counted to see if the number of people observed to fall into one category or the other is significant

REQUIRE

Original numbers (not percentages, etc.)
Data sets independent of each other
Ideally at least five expected frequencies
Simple chi-square table (p. 44)

RESULTS

The values of χ^2 must be equal to or greater than the value given in the table to be significant

METHOD

1 Place the data in a table format (similar to a spreadsheet) – the number in each cell is the observed frequency data (in this case A, B, C, D)

2 Total the data in each row and each column

A	B	A+B
C	D	C+D
A+C	B+D	A+B+C+D = N

3 Total the rows and columns to find N

4 Calculate the expected frequency (E) for each cell by multiplying the row total and the column total and dividing by N

5 For each cell, take the observed frequency (O) from the expected frequency (E) (or the expected frequency (E) from the observed frequency (O) if that is larger) and substract 0.5

6 Square the answer and divide by the expected frequency (E) for each cell

7 χ^2 = the total of the answers obtained in step **5** for each cell

8 Using the table read off the value of χ^2

Formula

$$\chi^2 = \sum \frac{(O - E - 0.5)^2}{E}$$

O = observed frequencies
E = expected frequencies
$\sum$ = sum of
0.5 = Yates correction

Example

You have observed a group of women selecting food in a canteen and obtain the following results

1 Place the data in table format

	Observed selecting salad Column A	Observed selecting chips Column B	Totals observed
Average weight Row C	230	275	505
Obese Row D	300	96	396
Totals	530	371	901 (N)

2 Total the data in each row and each column

3 Total the rows and columns to find $N = 901$

4 Calculate the expected frequency for each cell by multiplying the row total and the column total and dividing by N

expected frequency cell AC $= 505 \times 530 \div 901 = 297.06$

expected frequency cell BC $= 505 \times 371 \div 901 = 207.94$

expected frequency cell AD $= 396 \times 530 \div 901 = 232.94$

expected frequency cell BD $= 396 \times 371 \div 901 = 163.06$

5 For each cell, take the observed frequency from the expected frequency (or the expected frequency from the observed frequency if that is larger) and subtract 0.5

cell AC $= 297.06 - 230 - 0.5 = 66.56$

cell BC $= 275 - 207.94 - 0.5 = 66.56$

cell AD $= 300 - 232.94 - 0.5 = 66.56$

cell BD $= 163.06 - 96 - 0.5 = 66.56$

6 Square the answer and divide by the expected frequency for each cell

cell AC $= 66.56^2 \div 297.06 = 14.91$

cell BC $= 66.56^2 \div 207.94 = 21.30$

cell AD $= 66.56^2 \div 232.94 = 19.02$

cell BD $= 66.56^2 \div 163.06 = 27.17$

7 $\chi^2 = 14.91 + 21.30 + 19.02 + 27.17 = 82.40$

8 Using the table on page 44, read off the value of χ^2

As χ^2 is greater than the value (10.83) given in the table, the results of the test are significant

SIMPLE CHI-SQUARE: USING EXCEL

	A	B	C	D	E	F	G
1	230	275	= A1 + B1	A1 =	= A3* C1/C3	= E1 – A1 – 0.5	= F1^2/E1
2	300	96	= A2 + B2	A2 =	= A3* C2/C3	= A2 – E2 – 0.5	= F2^2/E2
3	= A1 + A2	= B1 + B2	= C1 + C2	B1 =	= B3* C1/C3	= B1 – E3 – 0.5	= F3^2/E3
4				B2 =	= B3* C2/C3	= E4 – B2 – 0.5	= F4^2/E4
5							= SUM (G1:G4)

Step 1 = A1, B1, A2, B2
Step 2 = A3, B3, C1 and C2
Step 3 = C3
Step 4 = E1 to E4
Step 5 = F1 to F4
Step 6 = G1 to G4
Step 7 = G5

The results in Excel are

	A	B	C	D	E	F	G
1	230	275	505	A1 =	297.06	66.56	14.91
2	300	96	396	A2 =	232.94	66.56	19.02
3	530	371	901	B1 =	207.94	66.56	21.30
4				B2 =	163.06	66.56	27.17
5							82.40

SIMPLE CHI-SQUARE TABLE

Level of significance for two-tailed tests		
0.1	0.05	0.01
2.71	3.84	6.64

21. Complex chi-square test (χ^2)

USE

To compare groups where their observed behaviour has been counted to see if the number of people observed to fall into one category or the other is significant

REQUIRE

Original numbers (not percentages, etc.)
Data sets independent of each other
Ideally at least five expected frequencies
Complex chi-square table (p. 51)

RESULTS

The values of χ^2 must be equal to or greater than the value given in the table to be significant

METHOD

1 Place the data in a table format (similar to a spreadsheet) – the number in each cell is the observed data (O)
2 Total the data in each row and each column

A	B	C	A+B+C
D	E	F	D+E+F
G	H	I	G+H+I
A+D+G	B+E+H	C+F+I	A+B+C+ D+E+F+G+H+ I =N

3 Total the rows and columns to find N
4 Calculate the expected frequency (E) for each cell by multiplying the row total and the column total and dividing by N

5 For each cell, take the observed frequency (O) from the expected frequency (E) (or the expected frequency (E) from the observed frequency (O) if that is larger)

6 Square the answer and divide by the expected frequency (E) for each cell

7 χ^2 = the total of the answers obtained in step **5** for each cell

8 Find *df* by taking the number of rows -1, multiplied by the number of columns -1

9 Using the table, read off the value of χ^2 at the appropriate level of *df*

Formula

$$\chi^2 = \sum \frac{(O - E)^2}{E}$$

O = observed frequencies
E = expected frequencies
$\sum$ = sum of

Example

You have observed a group of people selecting food in a canteen and obtain the following results

1 Place the data in table format

	Observed eating salad Column A	Observed eating chips Column B	Observed eating Fruit Column C	Totals observed
Men Row D	23	40	15	78
Women Row E	45	9	30	84
Children Row F	12	49	3	64
Totals	80	98	48	226 (N)

2 Total the data in each row and each column

3 Total the rows and columns to find $N = 226$

4 Calculate the expected frequency for each cell by multiplying the row total and the column total and dividing by N

expected frequency cell AD = $78 \times 80 \div 226 = 27.61$

expected frequency cell BD = $78 \times 98 \div 226 = 33.82$

expected frequency cell CD = $78 \times 48 \div 226 = 16.56$

expected frequency cell AE = $84 \times 80 \div 226 = 29.73$

expected frequency cell BE = $84 \times 98 \div 226 = 36.42$

expected frequency cell CE = $84 \times 48 \div 226 = 17.84$

expected frequency cell AF = $64 \times 80 \div 226 = 22.65$

expected frequency cell BF = $64 \times 98 \div 226 = 27.75$

expected frequency cell CF = $64 \times 48 \div 226 = 13.59$

5 For each cell, take the observed frequency from the expected frequency (or the expected frequency from the observed frequency if that is larger)

cell AD = $27.61 - 23 = 4.61$

cell BD = $40 - 33.82 = 6.18$

cell CD = $16.56 - 15 = 1.56$

cell AE = $45 - 29.73 = 15.27$

cell BE = $36.42 - 9 = 27.42$

cell CE = $30 - 17.84 = 12.16$

cell AF = $22.65 - 12 = 10.65$

cell BF = $49 - 27.75 = 21.25$

cell CF = $13.59 - 3 = 10.59$

6 Square the answer and divide by the expected frequency for each cell

cell AD $= 4.61^2 \div 27.61 = 0.77$

cell BD $= 6.18^2 \div 33.82 = 1.13$

cell CD $= 1.56^2 \div 16.56 = 0.15$

cell AE $= 15.27^2 \div 29.73 = 7.84$

cell BE $= 27.42^2 \div 36.42 = 20.64$

cell CE $= 12.16^2 \div 17.84 = 8.29$

cell AF $= 10.65^2 \div 22.65 = 5$

cell BF $= 21.25^2 \div 27.75 = 16.69$

cell CF $= 10.59^2 \div 13.59 = 8.25$

7 $\chi^2 = 0.77 + 1.13 + 0.15 + 7.84$
$+20.64 + 8.29 + 5 + 16.69 + 8.25 = 68.35$

8 Find *df*

$(3 - 1) \times (3 - 1) = 4$

9 Using the table on page 51, read off the value of χ^2 at the value of $df = 4$

10 As χ^2 is greater than the value given in the table, the results of the test are significant

COMPLEX CHI-SQUARE: USING A SPREADSHEET

From the previous example enter:

	A	B	C	D	E	F	G	H
1	23	40	15	= SUM(A1:C1)	A1=	= D1*A4/D4	= F1-A1	= G1^2/F1
2	45	9	30	= SUM(A2:C2)	B1=	= D1*B4/D4	= B1-F2	= G2^2/F2
3	12	49	3	= SUM(A3:C3)	C1=	= D1*C4/D4	= F3-C1	= G3^2/F3
4	= SUM (A1:A3)	= SUM(B1:B3)	= SUM(C1:C3)	= SUM(D1:D3)	A2=	= D2*A4/D4	= A2-F4	= G4^2/F4
5					B2=	= D2*B4/D4	= F5-B2	= G5^2/F5
6					C2=	= D2*C4/D4	= C2-F6	= G6^2/F6
7					A3=	= D3*A4/D4	= F7-A3	= G7^2/F7
8					B3=	= D3*B4/D4	= B3-F8	= G8^2/F8
9					C3=	= D3*C4/D4	= F9-C3	= G9^2/F9
10								= SUM (H1:H9)

Step 1 = A1-A3, B1-B3, C1-C3
Step 2 = A4, B4, C4, D1, D2 and D3
Step 3 = D4
Step 4 = F1 to F9
Step 5 = G1 to G9
Step 6 = H1 to H9
Step 7 = H10

The result in a spreadsheet is:

	A	B	C	D	E	F	G	H
1	23	40	15	78	A1 =	27.61	4.61	0.77
2	45	9	30	84	B1 =	33.82	6.18	1.13
3	12	49	3	64	C1 =	16.57	1.57	0.15
4	80	98	48	226	A2 =	29.73	15.27	7.84
5					B2 =	36.42	27.42	20.65
6					C2 =	17.84	12.16	8.29
7					A3 =	22.65	10.65	5.01
8					B3 =	27.75	21.25	16.27
9					C3 =	13.59	10.59	8.26
10								68.35

COMPLEX CHI-SQUARE TABLE

	Level of significance for one-tailed tests		
	0.05	0.025	0.005
	Level of significance for two-tailed tests		
df	0.1	0.05	0.01
1	2.71	3.84	6.64
2	4.60	5.99	9.21
3	6.25	7.82	11.35
4	7.78	9.49	13.28
5	9.24	11.07	15.09
6	10.65	12.59	16.81
7	12.02	14.07	18.48
8	13.36	15.51	20.09
9	14.68	16.92	21.67
10	15.99	18.31	23.21
11	17.28	19.68	24.72
12	18.55	21.03	26.22
13	19.81	22.36	27.69
14	21.06	23.69	29.14
15	22.31	25.00	30.58
16	23.54	26.30	32.00
17	24.77	27.59	33.41
18	25.99	28.87	34.80
19	27.20	30.14	36.19
20	28.41	31.41	37.57

22. Mann–Whitney *U* test

USE

For data measured using an ordinal scale

REQUIRE

Two sets of unmatched data
Table of values for U (p. 54)

RESULTS

If the values for U are less than the values in the table, the results are significant

METHOD

1 Count the number of scores in each set of results
2 Call the total number of scores in the smaller set N_A
3 Call the total number of scores in the larger set N_B
4 Rank the numbers of all the scores (i.e. of both sets together) *Ranking sets of scores p. 9*
5 Add the ranks in the smallest group $\sum R_A$
6 Calculate U using the formula:

$$U = N_A N_B + \frac{N_A(N_A + 1)}{2} - \sum R_A$$

7 Using the tables, calculate the significance of U

Example

Subject	A	B	Subject	A	B
1	6	2	**6**	9	2
2	4	9	**7**	7	4
3	7	3	**8**	3	9
4	4	8	**9**	6	4
5	6	1	**10**		4

1 Count the scores in each set of results

2 The number of scores in smallest set, $N_A = 9$

3 The number of scores in the largest set, $N_B = 10$

4 Ranking the scores *Ranking sets of scores p. 9*

Score	Rank	Score	Rank	Score	Rank	Score	Rank
1	**1**	4	**8**	6	**12**	8	**16**
2	**2.5**	4	**8**	6	**12**	9	**18**
2	**2.5**	4	**8**	6	**12**	9	**18**
3	**4.5**	4	**8**	7	**14.5**	9	**18**
3	**4.5**	4	**8**	7	**14.5**		

5 Add the ranks of the smallest group, $\sum R_A = 103.5$

6 Calculate U

$$= 9 \times 10 + \frac{9(9+1)}{2} - 103.5$$

$$= 90 + 45 - 103.5$$

$$= 31.5$$

7 Using the table, as U is greater than 20, the results are not significant

MANN–WHITNEY *U* TEST TABLE

The table gives the values for *U* for two-tailed tests at 0.05 significance
For one-tailed tests the values are at 0.025 significance
If the value of *U* is less than the number given on the table, the results are significant

N_B	N_A	5	6	7	8	9	10	11	12	13	14	15	16	17	18	19	20
5		2	3	5	6	7	8	9	11	12	13	14	15	17	18	19	20
6			5	6	8	10	11	13	14	16	17	19	21	22	24	25	27
7				8	10	12	14	16	18	20	22	24	26	28	30	32	34
8					13	15	17	19	22	24	26	29	31	34	36	38	41
9						17	20	23	26	28	31	34	37	39	42	45	48
10							23	26	29	33	36	39	42	45	48	52	55
11								30	33	37	40	44	47	51	55	58	62
12									37	41	45	49	53	57	61	65	69
13										45	50	54	59	63	67	72	76
14											55	59	64	69	74	78	83
15												64	70	75	80	85	90
16													75	81	86	92	98
17														87	93	99	105
18															99	106	112
19																113	119
20																	127

23. *t*-Test for related samples

USE

When comparing two sets of results, i.e. paired results

REQUIRE

Paired (matched) data
The sets of scores are normally distributed
The scores are on an interval scale
The scores have similar variances
t-Test table (p. 60)

RESULTS

If the value of t is equal to or greater than the value given in the table the results are significant

METHOD

1 Count the number of pairs of scores, N
2 Subtract 1 from N to find the degrees of freedom, df

Statistical glossary p. 66

3 Multiply N by df
4 Find the mean of each set of scores $\bar{x}$ and $\bar{y}$
5 Take the smaller value of $\bar{x}$ and $\bar{y}$ from the larger to get the difference between the means
6 Find the differences (D) for each pair of scores by taking each score in column 2 from its pair in column 1 to get values of D
7 Total the value of differences and square the answer to get $\sum D^2$

8 Add the values of D together (taking note of the signs) and square the answer to get $(\sum D)^2$

9 Divide $(\sum D)^2$ by N and take the answer from $\sum D$ and divide by $(N \times df)$

10 Find the square root of the answer to step **9** and divide the answer by the difference between the two means to obtain the value of t

11 Using the table, read off the value of t at the level of df

12 The answer calculated must be larger than or equal to the value in the table to be significant

Formula

The formula for the above calculation is:

$$t = \frac{|\bar{x} - \bar{y}|}{\sqrt{\dfrac{\sum D^2 - \dfrac{\left(\sum D\right)^2}{N}}{N(N-1)}}}$$

$||$ = absolute value, i.e. independent of the + or − sign
$\bar{x}$ = mean of list 1
$\bar{y}$ = mean of list 2
D = difference between the x and y scores
$\sum$ = sum of
N = total number of pairs of scores

Example

Subject	Rating X	Rating Y	Subject	Rating X	Rating Y
1	6	2	6	9	2
2	4	9	7	7	4
3	7	3	8	3	9
4	4	8	9	6	4
5	6	1	10	8	4

1 Count the number of pairs of scores, $N = 10$

2 Subtract 1 from N to find $df = 9$

3 Multiply N by $df = 90$

4 Find the mean of each set of scores $\bar{x}$ and $\bar{y}$

$x = 6 + 4 + 7 + 4 + 6 + 9 + 7 + 3 + 6 + 8 = 60 \div 10 = 6$

$y = 2 + 9 + 3 + 8 + 1 + 2 + 4 + 9 + 4 + 4 = 46 \div 10 = 4.6$

5 The difference between the means $= 6 - 4.6 = 1.4$

6 Take each score in column y from its pair in column x

$6 - 2 = 4,\ 4 - 9 = -5,\ 7 - 3 = 4,\ 4 - 8 = -4,$
$6 - 1 = 5,\ 9 - 2 = 7,\ 7 - 4 = 3,\ 3 - 9 = -6,$
$6 - 4 = 2,\ 8 - 4 = 4$

7 $\sum D^2 = 4^2 + -5^2 + 4^2 + -4^2 + 5^2 + 7^2 + 3^2 + -6^2 + 2^2 + 4^2 = 200$

8 $(\sum D)^2 = 4 + -5 + 4 + -4 + 5 + 7 + 3 + -6 + 2 + 4 = 14$
$14^2 = 196$

9 $(\sum D)^2 \div N = 196 \div 10 = 19.6$

$\sum D^2 - 19.6 = 200 - 19.6 = 180.4$
$N \times df = 90$
$180.4 \div 90 = 2.0044$

10 $t =$ difference between the means divided by $\sqrt{2.004} = 1.4 \div 1.416 = 0.989$

11 Using the table on page 60, read off the value of t at the level of $df = 9$, which is 2.262 at 0.05 level of significance for two-tailed tests

12 The answer calculated is lower than the reading on the table and therefore the results are not significant

t-TEST FOR RELATED SAMPLES: USING A SPREADSHEET

From the previous example enter:

	A	B	C	D	E	F
1	6	2	= A1 – B2	= C1^2		= A11 – B11
2	4	9	= A2 – B2	= C2^2		= C11/10
3	7	3	= A3 – B3	= C3^2		= D11 – F2
4	4	8	= A4 – B4	= C4^2		= F3/90
5	6	1	= A5 – B5	= C5^2		= F1/SQRT(F4)
6	9	2	= A6 – B6	= C6^2		
7	7	4	= A7 – B7	= C7^2		
8	3	9	= A8 – B8	= C8^2		
9	6	4	= A9 – B9	= C9^2		
10	8	4	= A10 – B10	= C10^2		
11	= SUM (A1:A10)/10	= SUM (B1:B10)/10	= SUM (C1:C10)^2	= SUM (D1:D10)		

Step 1 = 10
Step 2 = 9
Step 3 = 90
Step 4 = A11 and B11
Step 5 = F1

Step 6 = C1 to C10
Step 7 = D11
Step 8 = C11
Step 9 = F2, F3 and F4
Step 10 = F5

The result in the spreadsheet is:

	A	B	C	D	E	F
1	6	2	4	4		1.4
2	4	9	−5	25		19.6
3	7	3	4	16		180.4
4	4	8	−4	16		2.004
5	6	1	5	25		0.989
6	9	2	7	49		
7	7	4	3	9		
8	3	9	−6	36		
9	6	4	2	4		
10	8	4	4	16		
11	6	4.6	196	200		

t-TEST TABLE

Values of *t* for two-tailed tests
For one-tailed tests, divide the significance level by 2

Level of significance				Level of significance			
df	**0.10**	**0.05**	**0.02**	*df*	**0.10**	**0.05**	**0.02**
1	6.314	12.71	31.82	**18**	1.734	2.101	2.552
2	2.920	4.303	6.965	**19**	1.729	2.093	2.540
3	2.353	3.182	4.541	**20**	1.725	2.086	2.528
4	2.132	2.776	3.747	**21**	1.721	2.080	2.518
5	2.015	2.571	3.365	**22**	1.717	2.074	2.508
6	1.943	2.447	3.143	**23**	1.714	2.069	2.500
7	1.895	2.365	2.998	**24**	1.711	2.064	2.492
8	1.860	2.306	2.897	**25**	1.708	2.060	2.485
9	1.833	2.262	2.821	**26**	1.706	2.056	2.479
10	1.812	2.228	2.764	**27**	1.703	2.052	2.473
11	1.796	2.201	2.718	**28**	1.701	2.048	2.467
12	1.782	2.179	2.681	**29**	1.699	2.045	2.462
13	1.771	2.160	2.650	**30**	1.697	2.042	2.457
14	1.761	2.145	2.624	**40**	1.684	2.021	2.423
15	1.753	2.131	2.602	**60**	1.671	2.000	2.390
16	1.746	2.120	2.583	**120**	1.658	1.980	2.358
17	1.740	2.110	2.567	**240**	1.645	1.960	2.326

24. *t*-Test for unrelated samples

USE

For small samples

REQUIRE

Two sets of data (unmatched)
Scores on an interval scale
Scores that are normally distributed
Scores that have similar variances
t-Test table (p. 60)

RESULTS

If the value of t is equal to or greater than the value given on the table the results are significant

METHOD

1 Count the scores in each set N_A and N_B

2 $(N_A + N_B) \div N_A N_B = C$

3 Add the scores in list A, square the result $(\sum N_A)^2$

4 Divide $(\sum N_A)^2$ by $N_A = D$

5 Square the scores in list A and add them together $\sum N_A^2$ and take D from the result $= E$

6 Add the scores in list B, square the result $(\sum N_B)^2$

7 Divide $(\sum N_B)^2$ by $N_B = F$

8 Square the scores in list B and add them together $\sum N_B^2$ and take F from the result $= G$

9 $E + G = H$

10 Calculate df by $(N_A + N_B) - 2$

11 $(H \div df) \times C = J$

12 Find the $\sqrt{J} = K$

13 Find the mean of list A and the mean of list B and take the smaller from the larger $= L$

14 $L \div K = t$

15 Using the tables, read off the value of t at the level of df

16 The answer calculated must be larger than or equal to the value in the table to be significant

Formula

$$t = \frac{|\bar{A} - \bar{B}|}{\sqrt{\left\{\frac{\left(\sum N_A^2 - \frac{\left(\sum N_A\right)^2}{N_A}\right) + \left(\sum N_B^2 - \frac{\left(\sum N_B\right)^2}{N_B}\right)}{(N_A + N_B - 2)}\right\}\left\{\frac{N_A + N_B}{(N_A)(N_B)}\right\}}}$$

$\bar{A}$ = mean group A
$\bar{B}$ = mean group B
$\sum$ = sum of
N_A = number list A
N_B = number list B
$||$ = absolute value, i.e. independent of the + or − sign

Example

List A	List B
6	3
7	4
8	4
8	5
9	5
6	

1 $N_A = 6$, $N_B = 5$

2 $11 \div 30 = 0.367(C)$

3 Add the scores in list $A = 44$, square the result $= 1936$

4 Divide $(\sum N_A)^2$ by $N_A = 1936 \div 6 = 322.667(D)$

5 Square the scores in list A and add them together $= 330$ and take (D) from the result $= 7.333(E)$

6 Add the scores in list B $= 21$, square the result $(\sum N_B)^2 = 441$

7 Divide 441 by $5 = 88.2(F)$

8 Square the scores in list B and add them together $\sum N_B{}^2 = 91$ and take F from the result $= 2.8(G)$

9 $7.33 + 2.8 = 10.133(H)$

10 Calculate *df* by $(N_A + N_B) - 2 = 6 + 5 - 2 = 11 - 2 = 9$

11 $(10.13 \div 9) \times 0.36 = 0.413(J)$

12 Find the $\sqrt{J} = 0.643(K)$

13 Find the mean of list A $= 44 \div 6 = 7.333$ and the mean of list B $= 21 \div 5 = 4.2$ and take the smaller from the larger $= 3.133(L)$

14 $3.13 \div 0.636 = 4.87(t)$

15 Using the table on page 60, read off the value of t at the level of $df = 9$, $t = 1.833$

16 The answer calculated must be larger than or equal to the value in the table to be significant. Therefore the answer is significant

t-TEST FOR UNRELATED SAMPLES: USING A SPREADSHEET

	A	B	C	D	E	F
1	6	3	= A1^2	= B1^2		= (5 + 6)/5*6
2	7	4	= A2^2	= B2^2		= A8/6
3	8	4	= A3^2	= B3^2		= C8 – F2
4	8	5	= A4^2	= B4^2		= B8/5
5	9	5	= A5^2	= B5^2		= D8 – F4
6	6		= A6^2			F3 + F5
7						= 5 + 6 – 2
8	= SUM (A1:A6)^2	= SUM (B1:B5)^2	= SUM (C1:C6)	= SUM (D1:D5)		= (F6/F7)*A8
9	= SUM (A1:A6)/6	= SUM (B1:B5)/5	= A9–B9	= C9/F9		= SQRT(F8)

Step 1 A = 5, B = 7
Step 2 = F1
Step 3 = A8
Step 4 = F2
Step 5 = F3
Step 6 = B8
Step 7 = F4

Step 8 = F5
Step 9 = F6
Step 10 = F7
Step 11 = F8
Step 12 = F9
Step 13 = C9
Step 14 = D9

The result in a spreadsheet is:

	A	B	C	D	E	F
1	6	3	36	9		0.366667
2	7	4	49	16		322.6667
3	8	4	64	16		7.33333
4	8	5	64	25		88.2
5	9	5	81	25		2.8
6	6		36			10.13333
7						9
8	1936	441	330	91		0.41284
9	7.3333	4.2	3.13333	4.8765		0.642526

25. Statistical glossary

Actual scores each score has a real value

Correlation coefficient (*r*) a value between +1 (perfect positive correlation) and −1 (perfect negative correlation), 0 = no linear relationship

Degrees of freedom (*df*) the number of known numbers in a sample required to be able to find the missing number, e.g. if a total sample of five numbers = 20 you would need to know four numbers to be able to find the fifth. Therefore *df* would = 4

Frequency the number of times a particular value occurs

Hypothesis a theory that forms the basis for experimental work

Interval status when the numbers are ordinal and the steps between each number are of equal size

Nominal scale a number given to objects that are similar to each other, a method of classification

Non-parametric test No assumptions are made about the distribution of scores, the data is ordinal, the test is not powerful

Normally distributed a bell-shaped, normal distribution curve is produced when statistical results are plotted

Normal population a normal distribution curve is produced when the data is plotted

Null hypothesis presumes that the sets of data, produced in an experiment, will not differ from each other

One-tailed hypothesis (test) a theory that predicts a particular outcome

Ordinal scale the numbers allotted to the ranking or ordering data in a rough sequence

Parametric the scores are from a normal population, the data is interval and therefore the test is powerful

Pattern of distribution looks at the frequency that a qualitative result occurs

Population the pool of information from which statistics are drawn

Probability the likelihood that something is going to occur

Qualitative tests measure 'soft data' – feelings, opinions, etc.

Quantitative tests	measure actual, numerical results
Related	the data is matched – each sample has a matched sample with one or more variables in common
Sample	the data taken from part of a population
Significance	the numerical probability that the results of an experiment are meaningful
Tied numbers	results of the same value
Two-tailed hypothesis (test)	a theory that predicts an outcome but does not state which direction it will take
Unrelated	whole groups of data are roughly matched but the individual samples are not
Variables	factors that can influence a statistical experiment
Variance	a measure of dispersal around the mean – standard deviation is a measure of variance
Z	Normal distribution $= \frac{x-\bar{x}}{\mathrm{SD}}$ where $x =$ the score, $\bar{x} =$ the mean and SD $=$ the standard deviation
$\sum$	sum of

≤	less than or equal to
≥	greater than or equal to
||	absolute value, i.e. independent of the + or – sign

IN EXCEL

^2	the number squared
/	divide
AVERAGE	finds the average values
B1:B4	from cell B1 to cell B4
COUNT	calculates the number of cells containing numbers rather than text
MAX	finds the largest number in the cells indicated
MIN	finds the smallest number in the cells indicated
ROUND	calculates a number to a specific number of decimal points
SQRT	square root
SUM	adds the number

SECTION TWO
Practical exercises

3.78

0.378

0.0378

26. Drug dosages

TABLETS

Formula

$$\text{Number of tablets required} = \frac{\text{Strength tablets required}}{\text{Strength of tablet available}}$$

Example

A patient is prescribed 200 mg of a drug. The drug is available in 50 mg tablets

Strength of tablets required = 200 mg
Strength of tablet available = 50 mg

$$\frac{200}{50} = \frac{20}{5}$$
$$= 4$$

Fractions p. 151

Therefore the number of tablets required = 4

INJECTION

Formula

Volume required =

$$\frac{\text{Strength required}}{\text{Strength of solution available}} \times \text{volume of solution available}$$

Example

A patient is prescribed 60 mg of a drug. The drug is available in vials containing 300 mg in 10 ml

Strength required = 60 mg
Strength of solution available = 300 mg
Volume of solution available = 10 ml

$$\frac{60}{300} \times 10 = \frac{600}{300}$$

Fractions p. 154

$$\frac{600}{300} = \frac{6}{3}$$

$$= 2$$

Therefore the volume required = 2 ml

NB: For volumes larger than 1 ml use one decimal place
For volumes less than 1 ml use two decimal places in the calculation

PAEDIATRIC DOSAGES: SINGLE DOSE

Formula

$$\text{Single dose} = \frac{\text{Weight of child in kg} \times \text{recommended daily dosage}}{\text{Number of doses per day}}$$

Example

If the recommended daily dose is 60 mg per kg per day and the child is to receive 3 doses per day, calculate the size of a single dose if the child weighs 17 kg

Weight of child = 17 kg
Recommended daily dose = 60 mg
Number of doses per day = 3

$$\frac{17 \times 60}{3} = \frac{1020}{3}$$
$$= 340$$

Fractions p. 154

Therefore 340 mg per single dose is required

27. Diluting solutions

TO CALCULATE THE QUANTITY OF STOCK SOLUTION REQUIRED

Formula

$$\text{Quantity to be diluted} = \frac{\%\text{ strength required} \times \text{total volume required in ml}}{\%\text{ strength of stock}}$$

Example

If 3 litres of a 0.9% solution are required, what quantity of 18% stock solution will be required and how much water will it need to be diluted with?

$$\%\text{ strength required} = 0.9\%$$

Percentage p. 155

$$\text{Total volume required} = 3\text{ litres} \times 1000 = 3000\text{ ml}$$

$$\%\text{ strength of stock} = 18\%$$

Place value p. 138

$$\frac{0.9 \times 3000}{18} = \frac{2700}{18} = 150$$

Fractions p. 154

Therefore 150 ml of stock solution is required

TO CALCULATE THE QUANTITY OF WATER REQUIRED

Formula

Quantity of water = total volume required − quantity to be diluted

Total volume required = 3000 ml

Quantity to be diluted = 150 ml

3000 − 150 = 2850

Therefore 2850 ml of water is required

28. Drip infusions

RATES

Formula

$$\text{Drops per minute} = \frac{\text{Volume of fluid} \times \text{delivery rate}}{\text{Time in minutes}}$$

Example

Calculate the rate of the infusion (drops per minute) if 900 ml is required to be given over 5 hours using an infusion set that delivers at 15 drops per ml

Volume of fluid = 900 ml
Delivery rate = 15 drops per ml
Time in minutes = 5 hours × 60 = 300 minutes

$$\frac{900}{300} \times 15 = \frac{13500}{300}$$

$$= \frac{135}{3}$$

$$= 45$$

Fractions p. 154

Therefore the rate of the infusion will be 45 drops per minute

TIME

Formula

$$\text{Time in hours} = \frac{\text{Volume of fluid}}{\text{Drops per hour}} \times \text{delivery rate}$$

Example

Calculate the time taken for an infusion to be delivered if 900 ml is being given at a rate of 45 drops per minute using an infusion set that delivers at 15 drops per ml

Volume of fluid = 900 ml
Delivery rate of the set = 15 drops per ml
Drops per hour = 45 × 60

$$\frac{900 \times 15}{45 \times 60} = \frac{13500}{2700}$$
$$= \frac{135}{27}$$
$$= 5$$

Fractions p. 154

Therefore the time taken will be 5 hours

29. Converting weight

Stones	Kilograms
1	6.4
2	12.7
3	19.1
4	25.4
5	31.8
6	38.1
7	44.5
8	50.8
9	57.2
10	63.5
11	69.9
12	76.2
13	82.6
14	88.9
15	95.3
16	101.6
17	108.0
18	114.3
19	120.7
20	127.0

Pounds	Kilograms
1	0.5
2	0.9
3	1.4
4	1.8
5	2.3
6	2.7
7	3.2
8	3.6
9	4.1
10	4.5
11	5.0
12	5.4
13	5.9

TO CHANGE POUNDS TO KILOGRAMS

Example

To change 10 stone 7 pounds to kilograms. Using the tables:

10 stone = 63.5 kg
7 pounds = 3.2 kg

Therefore 63.5 + 3.2 = 66.7 kg

TO CHANGE KILOGRAMS TO STONES AND POUNDS

Example

To change 72 kg to pounds. Using the tables:

69.9 kg = 11 stone
72 – 69.9 = 2.1 kg
2.1 kg = 5 pounds

Therefore 72 kg = 11 stone 5 pounds

USING A CALCULATOR TO CONVERT WEIGHT

TO CHANGE POUNDS TO KILOGRAMS

First change the stones to pounds | × | 14 |

Then change the pounds to kilograms | ÷ | 2.2 |

Example

To change 8 stone 7 pounds to kilograms

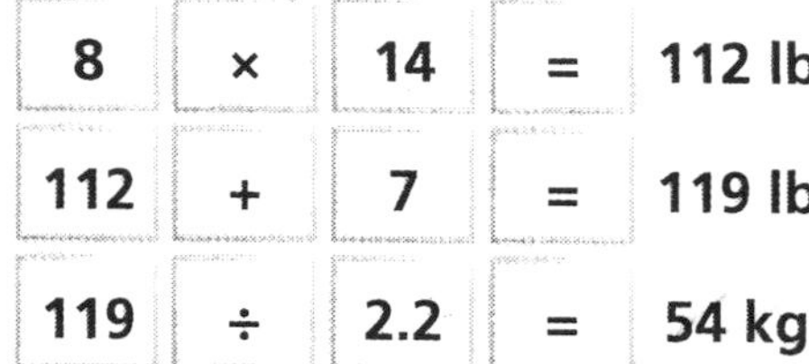
8 × 14 = 112 lb
112 + 7 = 119 lb
119 ÷ 2.2 = 54 kg

Therefore 8 stone 7 pounds = 54 kg

TO CHANGE KILOGRAMS TO STONES AND POUNDS

First change the kilograms to pounds | kg | × | 2.2 |

Then find out how many stones | lb | ÷ | 14 |

Next find the pounds | Numbers after the decimal point | × | 14 |

Example

To change 85 kg to stones and pounds

85	**×**	**2.2**	**=**	**187 lb**
187	**÷**	**14**	**=**	**13.3 stone**
0.3	**×**	**14**	**=**	**4.2 lb**

Therefore 85 kg = 13 stone 4 pounds

30. Surface area

NOMOGRAM FOR CALCULATING SURFACE AREAS

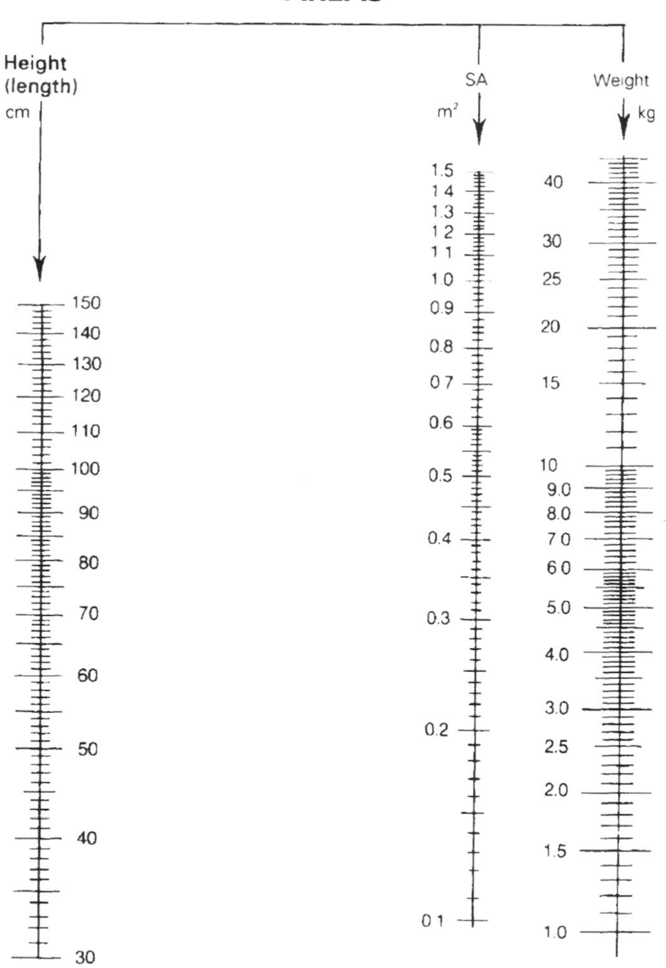

TO CALCULATE SURFACE AREA

Find the height and the weight of the child on the table. Join the two points with a straight line and where the line crosses the middle line read off the surface area (SA)

Example

A child who is 50 cm in height and weighs 20 kg will have a surface area of 0.58 m^2

←

The nomogram on page 84 is from Gatford J D, Anderson R E 1998 Nursing calculations, 5th edn, Churchill Livingstone, with permission.

31. Body mass index

Formula

$$\text{Body mass index} = \frac{\text{Body weight in kg}}{(\text{Height in metres})^2}$$

Example

A person is 1.7 metres in height and weighs 72 kg. Find their body mass

Weight = 72
Height = 1.7

$$\frac{72}{1.7^2} = \frac{72}{2.89}$$
$$= 24.9$$

Fractions p. 151
Indices p. 149

Therefore the body mass index = 25

32. Power

Formula

$$W = F \times d$$

$$p = \frac{W}{t}$$

W = mechanical work in joules
F = force in newtons
d = distance in metres
p = power in watts
t = time in seconds

Example

It takes a person 20 seconds to run up a 60 metre long hill. If the person exerts a force of 100 newtons:

a) How much work is done?

$$\begin{aligned} W &= F \times d \\ &= 100 \times 60 \\ &= 6000 \end{aligned}$$

Therefore the work done will be 6000 joules

b) How much power is generated?

$$\begin{aligned} P &= \frac{W}{t} \\ &= \frac{6000}{20} \\ &= 300 \end{aligned}$$

Fractions p. 154

Therefore the power generated will be 300 watts

33. Mechanical work

Formula

$$W = \left(\frac{1}{2}mv^2\right)_2 - \left(\frac{1}{2}mv^2\right)_1$$

W = mechanical work in joules
m = mass in kilograms
v = velocity in metres/second
$_1$ = start
$_2$ = end

Example

Calculate how much work is required to catch an object weighing 1.5 kg and travelling at 35 metres/second

$$W = (0.5\ mv^2)_2 - (0.5\ mv^2)_1$$

Indices p. 149

$$= (0.5 \times 1.5 \times 0 \times 0) - (0.5 \times 1.5 \times 35 \times 35)$$
$$= 0 - 918.75$$
$$= -918.75$$

Therefore the mechanical work done will be 918.75 joules

34. Speed

Formula

$$F \times t = (mv)_2 - (mv)_1$$

F = force in newtons
t = time in seconds
m = mass in kilograms
v = velocity in metres/second
$_1$ = start
$_2$ = end

Example

A person pushes an object weighing 50 kg for 10 seconds with a force of 90 newtons. Calculate the speed the object will have reached at the end of 10 seconds

BODMAS P. 136

$$\begin{aligned} F \times t &= (mv)_2 - (mv)_1 \\ 90 \times 10 &= (50 \times v) - (50 \times 0) \\ 900 &= (50 \times v) - 0 \\ v &= \frac{900}{50} \\ &= 18 \end{aligned}$$

Therefore the object will have reached a speed of 18 m/s

35. Velocity

Formulae

$$CE = PE + KE$$

$$PE = wt \times h$$

$$KE = \frac{1}{2} \times m \times v^2$$

CE = constant energy
PE = potential energy
KE = kinetic energy
wt = mass × gravity (g)
g = acceleration due to gravity (9.81 m/s^2)
h = height in metres
v = velocity is speed in a given direction in metres/second
m = mass in kg

Example 1

An object weighing 1.5 kg is dropped from a height of 2 metres. Calculate its velocity immediately before it hits the floor

$$CE = PE + KE$$

$$CE = (1.5 \times 9.81 \times 2) + (0)$$

$$CE = 29.43 \text{ joules}$$

$$29.43 = (0) + (0.5 \times m \times v^2)$$

Indices p. 149

$$29.43 = (0) + (0.5 \times 1.5 \times v^2)$$

$$v = \sqrt{\frac{29.43}{0.5 \times 1.5}}$$

Roots p. 150

$$= 3.43$$

Therefore the velocity of the object, immediately before it hits the floor, is 3.43 m/s

Example 2

If a ball weighing 10 kg is dropped from a height of 6 m, find the speed of the ball when it is 2 m above the floor

$$KE_1 + PE_1 = KE_2 + PE_2$$

$$0 + wt \times h = 1/2 \times m \times v^2 + wt \times h$$

$$10 \times 9.81 \times 6 = 1/2 \times 10 \times v^2 + 10 \times 9.81 \times 2$$

$$588.6 = 5 \times v^2 + 196.2$$

$$588.6 - 196.2 = 5 \times v^2$$

$$\sqrt{\frac{392.4}{5}} = v$$

Roots p. 150

$$v = 8.86$$

Therefore the speed of the ball is 8.86 m/s

36. Force–time graphs

Formulae

Area of a triangle $= \frac{1}{2}$ base $\times$ height

Area of a rectangle $=$ base $\times$ height

$$\frac{\text{Impulse}}{\text{mass}} = V - u$$

impulse = newtons times seconds
time = seconds
force = newtons
mass = kilograms
V = final velocity in metres per second
u = start velocity in metres per second

Example

From the force–time graph of a person weighing 75 kg starting from a stationary position, calculate:

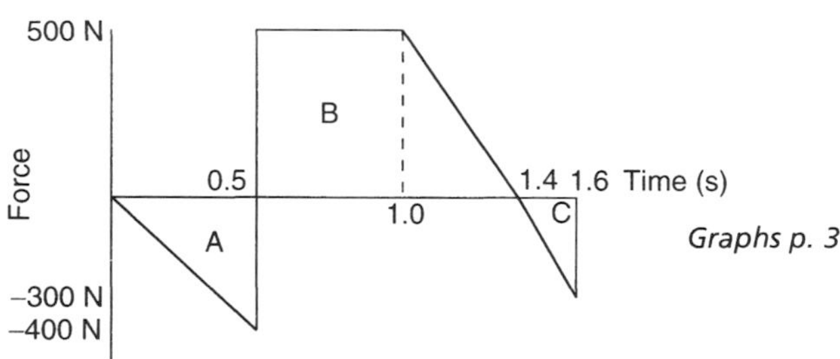

Graphs p. 3

a) The total impulse for the graph

Impulse A $= \frac{1}{2}$ base $\times$ height

$= 0.25 \times -400$ *Calculator glossary p. 165*

$= -100$ Ns

$$\begin{aligned}
\text{Impulse B} &= (\text{base} \times \text{height}) + (\tfrac{1}{2}\ \text{base} \times \text{height}) \\
&= (0.5 \times 500) + (\tfrac{1}{2} \times 0.4 \times 500) \\
&= 250 + 100 \\
&= 350\ \text{Ns}
\end{aligned}$$

$$\begin{aligned}
\text{Impulse C} &= \tfrac{1}{2}\ \text{base} \times \text{height} \\
&= \tfrac{1}{2} \times 0.2 \times -300 \\
&= -30\ \text{Ns}
\end{aligned}$$

$$\begin{aligned}
\text{Total impulse} &= \text{A} + \text{B} + \text{C} \\
&= -100 + 350 + -30 \\
&= 220
\end{aligned}$$

Therefore the total impulse is 220 Ns

b) The final velocity of the person

$$\frac{\text{Impulse}}{\text{mass}} = V - u$$

As the person started from a stationary position, $u = 0$

$$\begin{aligned}
\frac{220}{75} &= V \\
&= 2.9
\end{aligned}$$

Therefore the velocity is 2.9 m/s

37. Accelerated motion

Formulae

$$v = u + at$$

$$s = ut + \frac{1}{2}at^2$$

$$v^2 = u^2 + 2as$$

$$v = \frac{s}{t}$$

v = final velocity in metres per second
u = initial velocity in metres per second
a = acceleration in metres per second squared
t = time in seconds
s = displacement in metres

Example

A runner:

accelerates for 40 m at $1.5\,ms^{-2}$
runs at a constant velocity for $130\,ms^{-1}$
slows for 30 m at a rate of $-0.6\,ms^{-2}$

Calculate:

a) The time taken to run the first 40 m
NB: as the runner starts from a stationary position, $u = 0$

$$s = ut + \frac{1}{2}at^2$$

Equations equals signs p. 157

$$40 = 0 \times t + \tfrac{1}{2} \times 1.5 \times t^2$$

$$\sqrt{\frac{2 \times 40}{1.5}} = t$$

Roots p. 150

$$7.30 = t$$

Therefore the time taken to run the first 40 m is 7.30 s

b) The velocity after 40 m

$$v^2 = u^2 + 2as$$

Indices p. 149

$$v^2 = 0 + 2 \times 1.5 \times 40$$

$$v = \sqrt{120}$$

$$= 10.95\,\text{ms}^{-1}$$

Therefore the velocity after 40 m is 10.95 ms^{-1}

c) The time to cover the 130 m

$$v = \frac{s}{t}$$

$$10.95 = \frac{130}{t}$$

$$t = \frac{130}{10.95}$$

Equations equals signs p. 157

$$= 11.87$$

Therefore the time taken to travel 130 m is 11.87 s

d) The final velocity for the last 30 m

$$v^2 = u^2 + 2as$$

$$v^2 = 11.87^2 + 2 \times -0.6 \times 30$$

Indices p. 149

$$v^2 = 140.90 + (-36)$$

$$v = \sqrt{104.90}$$

$$= 10.24$$

Roots p. 150

Therefore the velocity for the final 30 m is $10.24\,\text{ms}^{-1}$

e) The time to cover the last 30 m

$$v = u + at$$

$$10.24 = 11.87 + (-0.6 \times t)$$

$$\frac{10.24 - 11.87}{-0.6} = t$$

Equations equals signs p. 157

$$2.72 = t$$

Therefore the time to cover the last 30 m is 2.72 s

38. Acceleration

Formula

$$a = \frac{v - u}{t}$$

a = acceleration in metres per second squared
u = start velocity in metres per second
v = end velocity in metres per second
t = time in seconds

Example

A football starts to roll at a speed (velocity) of 6 m/s. If the ball slows at the rate of $-0.4\,\text{ms}^{-2}$ how long will it take for it to stop?

$$a = \frac{v - u}{t}$$

$$-0.4 = \frac{0 - 6}{t}$$

Equations equals signs p. 157

$$t = \frac{0 - 6}{-0.4}$$

$$= 15$$

Therefore the ball will take 15 s to stop

ANGULAR ACCELERATION

Formula

$$\alpha = \frac{w_2 - w_1}{t}$$

α = angle of acceleration in radians per second squared
w_2 = end angle of velocity in radians per second
w_1 = start angle velocity in radians per second
t = time in seconds

$$1 \text{ radian} = \frac{360^\circ}{2\pi} = 57.3^\circ$$

Circles p. 138

$$\pi = 3.142$$

Example

A golfer has a swing with an average angular acceleration of 1.3 rad/s^2. Calculate the angle of velocity when they hit the ball after a 0.6 second swing
NB: as the swing starts from a stationary position, $w_1 = 0$

$$\alpha = \frac{w_2 - w_1}{t}$$

$$1.3 = \frac{w_2 - 0}{0.6}$$

Equations equals sign p. 157

$$1.3 \times 0.6 = w_2$$

$$0.78 = w_2$$

Therefore the angle of velocity is 0.78 rad/s

To change the answer to degree-based units:

$$= 0.78 \times 57.3$$

$$= 44.69 \text{ deg/s}$$

Therefore the angle of velocity is 44.69 degrees per second

39. Newton's law of motion

Formulae

$$F = m \times a \text{ (in a normal direction)}$$

$$F = T_1 + wt$$

$$F = T_2 + wt \times \sin\theta$$

$$F = T_3 + 0$$

$$F = T_4 - wt$$

$$a = \frac{v^2}{r}$$

F = force in newtons
m = mass in kilograms
a = acceleration in metres per second squared
wt = weight force = mass times 9.81 in newtons
T_1 = vertical force above the centre in newtons
T_2 = force at an angle to the centre in newtons
T_3 = horizontal force in newtons
T_4 = vertical force below the centre in newtons
sin = sine of the angle
v = velocity in metres per second
r = radius

Example

A person weighing 55 kg is swinging round an exercise bar at a constant speed of 6 m/s. The centre of gravity of the person is located 1 metre from the bar.

Find the force on the person's arms at the positions shown in the diagram:
Angle $\theta = 45^\circ$

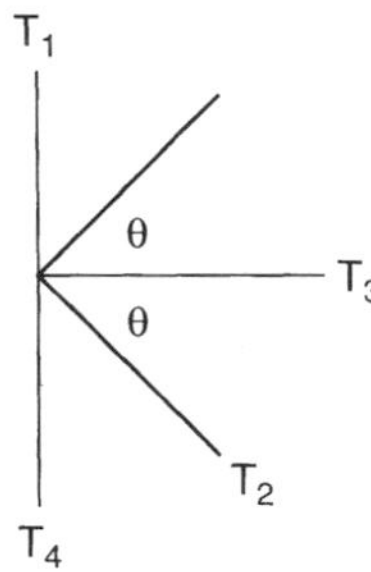

NB:

$$a = \frac{v^2}{r}$$

Indices p. 149

$$a = \frac{6^2}{1}$$
$$= 36\,\mathrm{m/s^2}$$

$$\begin{aligned} T_1 + wt &= m \times a \\ T_1 + 55 \times 9.81 &= 55 \times 36 \\ &= 1980 - 539.55 \\ &= 1440.45 \end{aligned}$$

Therefore the force at T_1 is 1440.45 N

$$T_2 + wt \times \sin\theta = m \times a$$

Triangles pp. 142–144

$$T_2 + (55 \times 9.81 \times \sin 45) = 55 \times 36$$

$$\mathrm{T}_2 = 1980 - 381.52$$

$$= 1598.48$$

Equations equals sign p. 157

Therefore the force at T_2 is 1598.48 N

$$T_3 + 0 = m \times a$$

$$T_3 = 55 \times 36$$

$$= 1980$$

Therefore the force at T_3 is 1980 N

$$T_4 - \mathrm{wt} = m \times a$$

$$\mathrm{T}_4 - 55 \times 9.81 = 55 \times 36$$

$$T_4 = 1980 + 539.55$$

$$= 2519.55$$

Therefore the force at T_4 is 2519.55 N

40. Dynamic equilibrium

Formula

$$F_v = (wt + F) - (m \times a)$$

F_v = vertical forces = 0
wt = weight force in newtons
F = force in newtons
m = mass = weight force ÷ 9.81 in kilograms
a = acceleration in metres per second squared

Example

A person of 570 N jumps from an aeroplane and is accelerating at $-9.2\,\text{m/s}^2$. How much drag is acting on the person prior to their parachute opening?

Equations equals sign p. 157

$$F_v = (-wt + F) - (m \times a)$$

$$0 = (-570 + F) - \left(\frac{570}{9.81} \times -9.2\right)$$

$$= (-570 + \text{F}) - (-534.56)$$

$$570 - 534.56 = F$$

Calculator glossary p. 165

$$35.44 = F$$

Therefore the drag is 35.44 N

41. Momentum

Formulae

$$p_1 = m \times v_1$$

$$\mathbf{F} \times \Delta t = \mathbf{p}_2 - \mathbf{p}_1$$

$$1\,\text{km/h} = 0.2778\,\text{m/s}$$

$\mathbf{p}_1$ = start momentum in kilograms metre per second
m = mass in kilograms
v_1 = velocity in metres per second
$\mathbf{F}$ = force in vector form, newtons
Δt = time interval in seconds
$\mathbf{p}_2$ = end momentum in kilograms metre per second
km/h = kilometres per hour
m/s = metres per second

Example

In a laboratory, a model weighing 70 kg and wearing a seat belt, travels at 90 km/hour. The model is stopped in 0.2 s.

Assuming there are no frictional forces, calculate the horizontal force applied to the seat belt when the model stops

$$1\,\text{km/h} = 0.2778\,\text{m/s}$$
$$90 = 90 \times 0.2778$$
$$= 25\,\text{m/s}$$

$$\mathbf{p}_1 = m \times v_1$$
$$= 70 \times 25$$
$$= 1750\,\text{kg.m/s}$$

As the model is stationary at the end, $\mathbf{p}_2 = 0$

$$\mathbf{F} \times \Delta t = \mathbf{p}_2 - \mathbf{p}_1$$

$$\mathbf{F} \times 0.2 = 0 - 1750$$

Equations equals sign p. 157

$$= \frac{-1750}{0.2}$$

$$= -8750 \text{ N applied to the model by the seat belt}$$

Therefore the horizontal force applied to the seat belt by the model is 8750 N

42. Moments

Formula

$$\frac{[(F_1' - F_1) + (F_2' - F_2)] \times I}{\text{wt}} = X \text{ or } Y$$

F' = initial force in newtons
F = final force in newtons
I = length in metres
X or Y = co-ordinates of the centre of mass
wt = weight force = mass × 9.81 in newtons

Example

A reaction board has an initial reading of 200 N. Calculate the *X* and *Y* position for the centre of mass for a person, weighing 65 kg lying on a rectangular reaction board

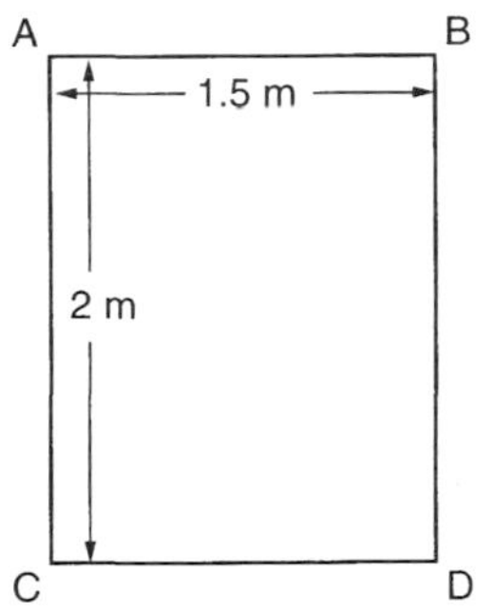

Final readings are A = 500 N
B = 450 N
C = 425 N
D = 300 N

Take moments round A and C

$$\frac{[(A' - A) + (C' - C)] \times I}{wt} = X$$

$$\frac{[(500 - 200) + (425 - 200)] \times 1.5}{65 \times 9.81} = X$$

BODMAS p. 136

$$\frac{525 \times 1.5}{637.65} = 1.24$$

Therefore $X = 1.24$ metres

If the moments are taken round B and D

$$\frac{[(B' - B) + (D' - D)] \times I}{wt} = X$$

$$\frac{[(450 - 200) + (300 - 200)] \times 1.5}{65 \times 9.81} = X$$

$$\frac{350 \times 1.5}{637.65} = 0.82$$

Therefore $X = 0.82$ metres

Therefore the moments around X are 1.24 m and 0.82 m

Take moments round A and B

$$\frac{[(A' - A) + (B' - B)] \times I}{wt} = Y$$

$$\frac{[(500 - 200) + (450 - 200)] \times 2.0}{65 \times 9.81} = Y$$

$$\frac{550 \times 2.0}{637.65} = 1.73$$

Therefore $Y = 1.73$ metres

If the moments are taken round C and D

$$\frac{[(C' - C) + (D' - D)] \times I}{wt} = Y$$

$$\frac{[(425 - 200) + (300 - 200)] \times 2.0}{65 \times 9.81} = Y$$

$$\frac{325 \times 2.0}{637.65} = 1.02$$

Therefore Y = 1.02 metres

Therefore the moments around *Y* are 1.73 m and 1.02 m

43. Force

Formula

$$\sum T = (F_1 \times d_1) - (F_2 \times d_2)$$

$\sum$ = sum of
T = torque
F = force in newtons
d = distance in metres

Example

How much force must be produced by a muscle 5 cm from the centre of rotation to support a weight of 65 N placed 25 cm away from the centre of rotation?

$$\sum T = (F_1 \times d_1) - (F_2 \times d_2)$$

BODMAS p. 136

As there is no movement, $\sum T = 0$

$$0 = (F_1 \times 0.05) - (65 \times 0.25)$$

$$= (0.05\ \mathrm{F}_1) - 16.25$$

Equations equals sign p. 157

$$\frac{16.25}{0.05} = F_1$$

$$325 = F_1$$

Therefore the force required is 325 N

FORCE APPLIED TO A PERSON

Formulae

$$\text{Sine} = \frac{\text{Opposite}}{\text{Hypotenuse}}$$

$$\text{Cosine} = \frac{\text{Adjacent}}{\text{Hypotenuse}}$$

Example

A force of 5.2 kN is applied to a footballer's leg at an angle of 30° to the horizontal. Calculate the vertical and horizontal components

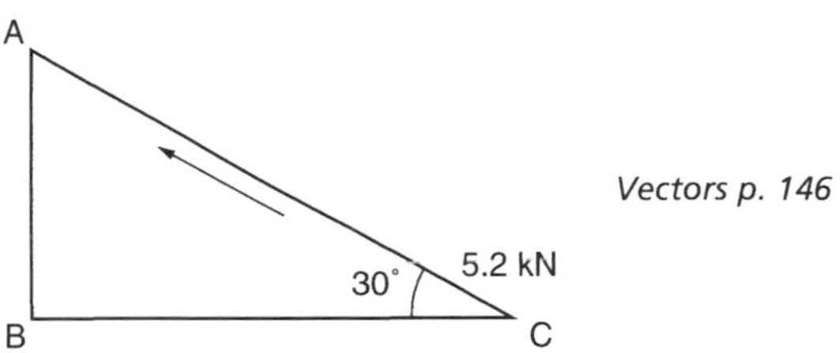

Vectors p. 146

To find the vertical force:

Triangles p. 142

$$\sin \text{ACB} = \frac{\text{AB}}{\text{AC}}$$

$$\text{AB} = \text{AC} \times \sin \text{ACB}$$

$$= 5.2 \times \sin 30^\circ$$

Therefore the vertical force AB = 2.6 kN

To find the horizontal force:

$$\cos ACB = \frac{BC}{AC}$$

Triangles p. 142

$$BC = AC \times \cos ACB$$
$$= 5.2 \times \cos 30^\circ$$

Therefore the horizontal force AB = 4.5 kN

FORCE APPLIED BY A PERSON

Formulae

$$\text{Sine} = \frac{\text{Opposite}}{\text{Hypotenuse}}$$

$$\text{Cosine} = \frac{\text{Adjacent}}{\text{Hypotenuse}}$$

Example

A force of 7.2 kN is applied through a footballers foot AC when it is at an angle of 42° to the ground. Resolve the resultant forces

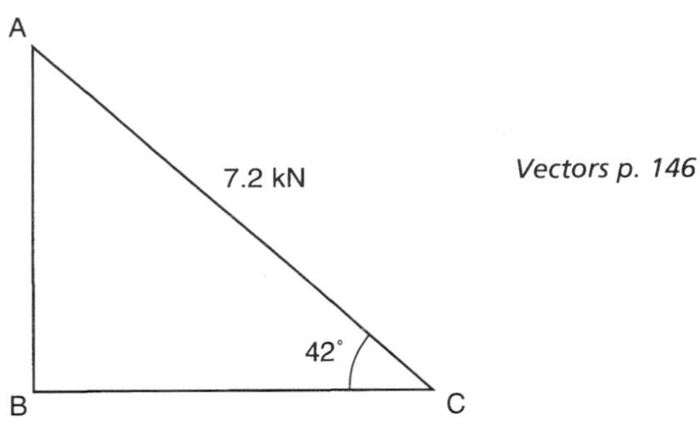

Vectors p. 146

To find the vertical force:

Triangles p. 142

$$\sin ACB = \frac{AB}{AC}$$

$$AB = AC \times \sin ACB$$

$$= 7.2 \times \sin 42^\circ$$

Therefore the vertical force AB = 4.8 kN

To find the horizontal force:

$$\cos ACB = \frac{BC}{AC}$$

Triangles p. 142

$$BC = AC \times \cos ACB$$

$$= 7.2 \times \cos 42^\circ$$

Therefore the horizontal force AB = 5.4 kN

HORIZONTAL FORCE

Formulae

$$\sum T = (F_1 \times d_1) - (F_2 \times d_2)$$

$$\text{Sine} = \frac{\text{Opposite}}{\text{Adjacent}}$$

T = torque
F = force in newtons
d = distance in metres

Example

Two people are standing on either side of a gate. Person 1 pushes the gate with a force of 40 **N**, 55 cm from the hinge at an angle of 30°. What force will person 2 need to apply if they push the gate at an angle of 90°, 45 cm from the hinge to prevent the gate from moving?

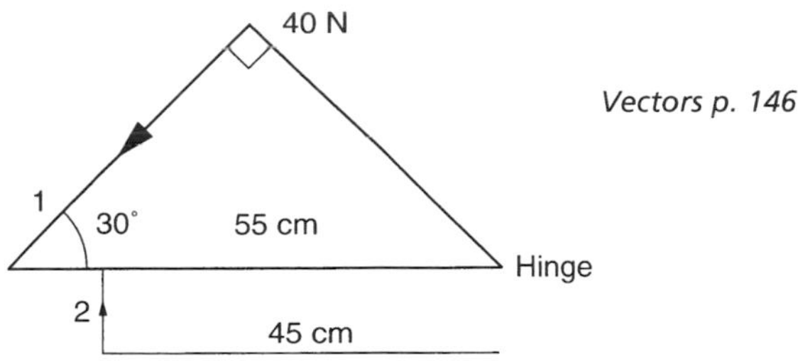

Vectors p. 146

Distance between person 1 and the hinge:

$$\sin 30^\circ = \frac{\text{distance person 1}}{\text{hypotenuse}}$$
$$= 0.55 \times \sin 30^\circ$$
$$= 0.275$$

Triangles p. 142

$$\sum T = (F_1 \times d_1) - (F_2 \times d_2)$$

BODMAS p. 136

As there is no movement, $\sum T = 0$

$$\begin{aligned} 0 &= (F_1 \times d_1) - (F_2 \times d_2) \\ &= (40 \times 0.275) - (F_2 \times 0.45) \\ &= 11 - (F_2 \times 0.45) \end{aligned}$$

Equations equals sign p. 157

$$\begin{aligned} F_2 &= \frac{11}{0.45} \\ &= 24.44 \end{aligned}$$

Therefore a force of 24.44 newtons will be required to prevent the gate from moving

VARYING FORCE

Formulae

$$W = A$$

$$\text{Area of a triangle} = \frac{1}{2}\ \text{base} \times \text{height}$$

$$\text{Area of a rectangle} = \text{base} \times \text{height}$$

$$\text{Area under a curve} = \int_{x_1}^{x_2} F \times dx$$

$$\text{Force with varying size} = \int_{x_1}^{x_2} c\sqrt{x} \times dx$$

W = work in joules
A = area in metres^2
x_1 = start of the displacement
x_2 = end of the displacement
F = force in newtons
c = constant of proportionality

Example 1

Calculate the work done in moving the object YZ in the diagram 18 metres to the right

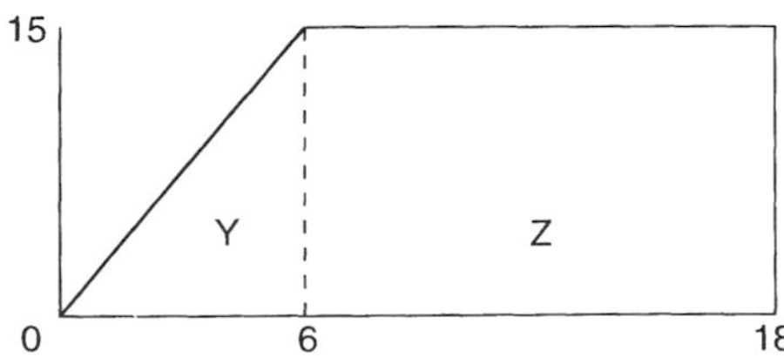

$$\text{Area of a triangle Y} = \frac{1}{2}\text{base} \times \text{height}$$
$$= \frac{1}{2} \times 6 \times 15$$
$$= 45$$

$$\text{Area of a rectangle Z} = \text{base} \times \text{height}$$
$$= 12 \times 15$$
$$= 180$$

$$W = \text{Area Y} + \text{Area Z}$$
$$= 45 + 180$$
$$= 225$$

Therefore the work done to move the object 18 metres is 225 joules

Example 2

Calculate the work done if a force of 50 newtons displaces a block a distance of 15 metres

$$W = \text{Area under the curve}$$
$$W = \int_{x_1}^{x_2} F \times dx$$

Calculus p. 163

$$W = \int_{0}^{15} 50 \times dx$$
$$W = [50x]_0^{15}$$
$$= (50 \times 15) - (50 \times 0)$$
$$= 750$$

Therefore the work done is 750 joules

Example 3

A force of varying size moves an object 16 metres and the following curve of force F against displacement x is plotted

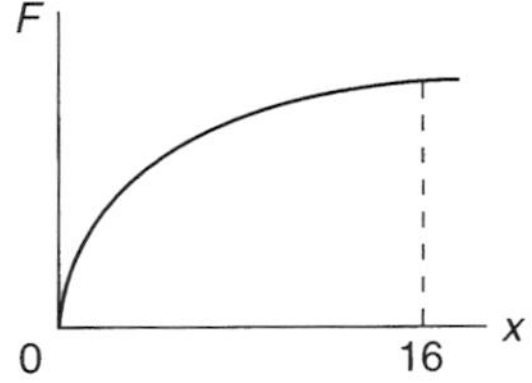

Calculate the work done if the constant of proportionality is 6

$$\text{Force with varying size} = \int_{x_1}^{x_2} c \times \sqrt{x} \times dx$$

$$= \int_0^{16} 6 \times x^{1/2} \times dx$$

$$= 6\left[\frac{x^{3/2}}{3/2}\right]_0^{16}$$

$$= \frac{2}{3} \times 6[16^{3/2} - 0^{3/2}]$$

$$= \frac{2}{3} \times 6[(\sqrt{16})^3 - 0]$$

$$= \frac{2}{3} \times 6 \times 4^3$$

$$= 256$$

Calculator glossary p. 165

Therefore the work done is 256 joules

44. Displacement

Formulae

$$\text{Pythagoras}: AC^2 = AB^2 + BC^2$$

$$\text{Tan BAC} = \frac{\text{Opposite}}{\text{Adjacent}}$$

$$\text{Cos BAC} = \frac{\text{Adjacent}}{\text{Hypotenuse}}$$

Example

A person is to swim from one side of a 100 m wide river to the other at a rate of 1.75 metres per second. There is a current flowing at the rate of 0.6 metres per second:

a) What will be the swimmer's total velocity?

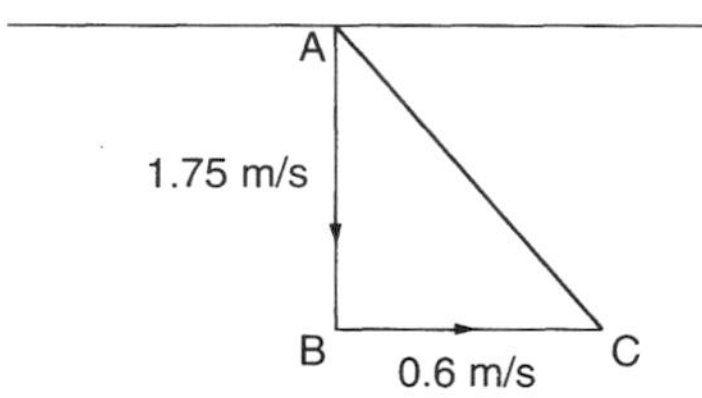

To find AC:

Triangles p. 142

$$AC^2 = AB^2 + BC^2$$

$$AC^2 = 1.75^2 + 0.6^2$$

$$= 3.06 + 0.36$$

$$= 3.42$$

$$AC = \sqrt{3.42} = 1.85$$

Therefore the resultant velocity will be 1.85 m/s

b) How far will they have to swim?

To find angle BAC:

Indices p. 149

Triangles p. 142

Calculator glossary p. 166

$$\tan \text{BAC} = \frac{\text{BC}}{\text{AB}}$$

$$= \frac{0.6}{1.75}$$

$$\tan \text{BAC} = 0.3429$$

$$\text{BAC} = \tan^{-1}(0.3429)$$

$$\text{BAC} = 18.9268^\circ$$

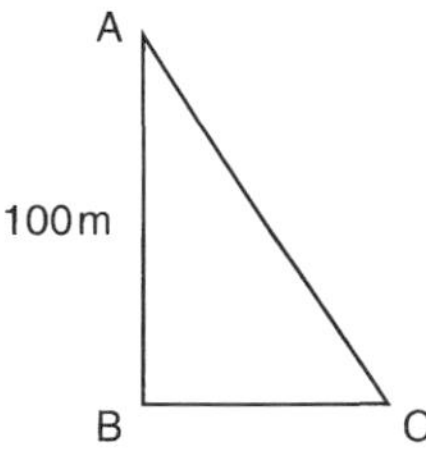

Triangles p. 142

$$\cos \text{BAC} = \frac{\text{Adjacent}}{\text{Hypotenuse}}$$

$$\cos \text{BAC} = \frac{\text{AB}}{\text{AC}}$$

Equations equals sign p. 157

$$\text{AC} = \frac{100}{\cos 18.9268^\circ}$$

$$= \frac{100}{0.9457}$$

$$= 105.72$$

Therefore they will have to swim 105.72 m

45. Torque

Formula

$$T = (F_1 \times d_1) - (F_2 \times d_2)$$

T = torque

F = force in newtons

d = distance in metres

Example

A board is placed on a fulcrum with an object placed on either end. Object 1 exerts a force of 180 N and is placed 1.4 metres from the fulcrum.

Object 2 exerts a force of 200 N and is placed 1.3 metres from the fulcrum.

Which object will drop to the ground?

$$T = (F_1 \times d_1) - (F_2 \times d_2)$$

$$T = (180 \times 1.4) - (200 \times 1.3)$$

BODMAS p. 136

$$= 252 - 260$$

$$= -8$$

Therefore as the result is in a negative direction, object 2 will fall

46. Coefficient of restitution

Formula

$$e = \sqrt{\frac{h_b}{h_d}}$$

e = coefficient of restitution

h_b = height of bounce in metres

h_d = height of drop in metres

Example

If a ball is dropped from a height of 1.5 metres and the coefficient of restitution is 0.9, how high will the ball bounce?

$$e = \sqrt{\frac{h_b}{h_d}}$$

Roots p. 150

$$0.9 = \sqrt{\frac{h_b}{1.5}}$$

Square both sides of the equation:

$$0.9^2 = \frac{h_b}{1.5}$$

$$h_b = 0.81 \times 1.5$$

$$= 1.22 \text{ m}$$

Therefore the height of the bounce will be 1.22 metres

47. Sensitometry

AVERAGE GRADIENT

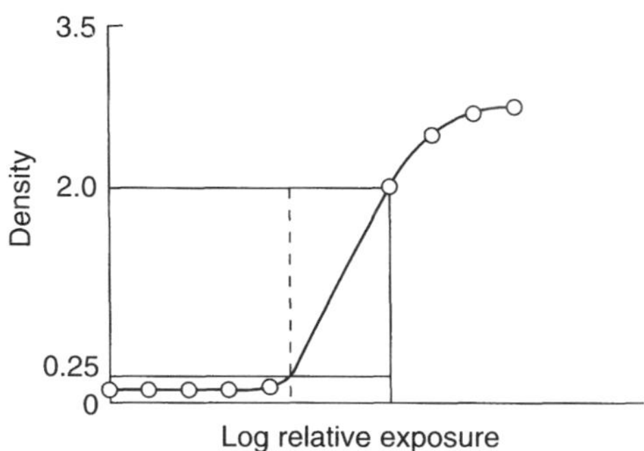

Formula

$$\text{Average gradient} = \frac{\text{Density } 2.0 - \text{Density } 0.25}{\text{Log exposure at D } 2.0 - \text{Log exposure at D } 0.25}$$

CONTRAST

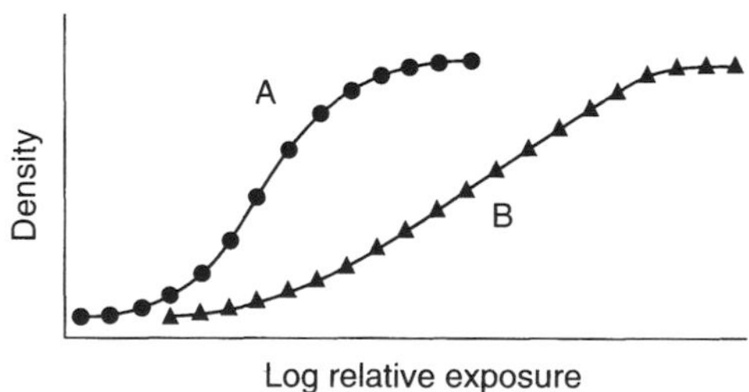

The steeper the gradient the greater the contrast

Example
Film A has a higher contrast than film B

SPEED
The nearer the Y axis the faster the film

Example
Film A is faster than film B

48. Exposure factors

kVp

Formulae

For film–screen combinations

$$\frac{\text{New kVp}^4}{\text{Old kVp}^4} = \frac{\text{Old mAs}}{\text{New mAs}} = \frac{\text{Old time}}{\text{New time}}$$

For direct exposure film

$$\frac{\text{New kVp}^2}{\text{Old kVp}^2} = \frac{\text{Old mAs}}{\text{New mAs}} = \frac{\text{Old time}}{\text{New time}}$$

kVp = kilovoltage peak
mAs = milliamperes per second

Example

If a radiograph was taken using 60 kVp, 200 mA and 0.4 seconds using a film screen combination, what kVp would be required if the time was reduced to 0.05 seconds, keeping the mAs the same?

Old kVp = 60
Old time = 0.4
New time = 0.05

Indices p. 149

$$\text{New kVp}^4 = \text{old kVp}^4 \times \frac{\text{Old time}}{\text{New time}}$$

$$\text{New kVp}^4 = 60^4 \times \frac{0.4}{0.05} = 60^4 \times 8$$

Equations equals sign p. 157

Taking the fourth root of both sides of the equation:

$$\text{New kVp} = \sqrt[4]{8} \times 60$$
$$= 100.9$$

Roots p. 150

Therefore the new kVp required is 100 kVp

CHANGING INTENSIFYING SCREENS

Formula 1

$$\text{New mAs} = \frac{\text{Old mAs}}{\text{Relative speed of the new system}}$$

mAs = milliamperes per second
FFD = focus, film distance

Example

A new screen film combination is introduced into an Imaging Department and is found to be three times faster than the original system. How would the following exposure factors be changed to give the same image using the new system?

kVp = 60
mAs = 10
FFD = 90 cm
Old mAs = 12
Relative speed = 3

$$\text{New mAs} = \frac{12}{3}$$
$$= 4 \text{ mAs}$$

Therefore the new mAs is 4 mAs

Formula 2

$$\text{Relative speed} = \frac{\text{New IF}}{\text{Old IF}}$$

IF = intensification factor

Example

A department has intensifying screens with an IF of 90 and has ordered new screens with an IF of 45. How does the speed of the new screens compare with that of the old ones?

New IF = 45
Old IF = 90

$$\text{Relative speed} = \frac{45}{90} = \frac{1}{2} = 0.5$$

Therefore the new screen combination is 0.5 times slower than the original screens

mAs

Formula

$$\text{mAs} = \text{mA} \times \text{time}$$

To achieve the same result but with a shorter time

$$\text{New mA} = \frac{\text{Original mAs}}{\text{New time}}$$

mAs = milliamperes per second
mA = milliamperes

Example

If the original mA was 200 with a time of 0.3 seconds, what mA would be required to maintain the same density if the time was reduced to 0.05 seconds?

Original mAs = 200 × 0.3
New time = 0.05

$$\frac{200 \times 0.3}{0.05} = 1200\,\text{mA}$$

Therefore the new mA = 1200 mA

FOCUS–FILM DISTANCE

Formula

$$\frac{\text{New mAs}}{\text{Old mAs}} = \frac{\text{New FFD}^2}{\text{Old FFD}^2}$$

mAs = milliamperes per second
FFD = focus film distance in cm

Example

A radiographer had taken a film at 60 kVp, 6 mAs at 120 cm. A follow-up radiograph is required but it is only possible to have an FFD of 100 cm. Calculate the mAs required to produce a radiograph of similar density to the first

Old mAs = 6
Old FFD = 120
New FFD = 100

$$\text{New mAs} = \frac{100^2 \times 6}{120^2}$$

Indices p. 149

$$= \frac{100 \times 100 \times 6}{120 \times 120}$$

$$\cong 4\,\text{mAs}$$

Therefore the new mAs is about 4 mAs

GRID FACTOR

Formula 1

New mAs with grid = Old mAs without a grid × grid factor

mAs = milliamperes per second

Example

A film was taken using 60 kVp, 12 mAs at 90 cm FFD and it was decided that the film needed repeating using a grid with a grid factor of 4:1. Calculate the new exposure factors required

Old mAs = 12
Grid factor = 4

$$\text{New mAs} = 12 \times 4$$
$$= 48\,\text{mAs}$$

Therefore the new mAs = 48 mAs

Formula 2

$$\text{mAs with new grid} = \frac{\text{New grid factor} \times \text{mAs with old grid}}{\text{Old grid factor}}$$

mAs = milliamperes per second

Example

If old grids with a grid factor of 9:1 were being replaced with new grids with a grid factor of 3:1 at 80 kVp, by how much will the new mAs need to be changed if the previous exposure factors were 80 kVp, 30 mAs at 90 cm FFD?

$$\text{New grid factor} = 3$$
$$\text{Old grid factor} = 9$$
$$\text{mAs with old grid} = 30$$
$$\text{mAs with new grid} = \frac{3 \times 30}{9}$$
$$= 10\,\text{mAs}$$

Therefore the mAs with the new grid = 10 mAs

SECTION THREE
Factors and formulae

3.78

0.378

0.0378

49. Checking your calculator

Before doing complex calculations on a calculator a check needs to be made to ensure that you are using a scientific calculator. To do this, key in:

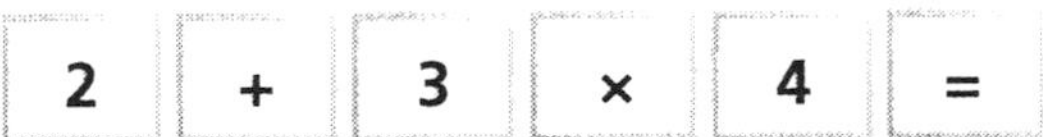

If you get the answer 14 then you have a scientific calculator and therefore can usually key in figures on one line in the order that they appear in the calculation

If you get the answer 20 you have not got a scientific calculator and you will have to key in the numbers in the same order that you would use if you were working the calculation out without using a calculator

50. Order of working

When working out more complex calculations you need to follow a particular order of working to get the correct answer. The order can be remembered by memorising the term **BODMAS**. This stands for:

B = Brackets
O = Of
D = Division
M = Multiplication
A = Addition
S = Subtraction

Therefore, to work out the sum:

$2 + 3 \times 4$

The multiplication is done first. Therefore:

$3 \times 4 = 12$
$+2 = 14$

51. Multiplication square

1	2	3	4	5	6	7	8	9	10
2	4	6	8	10	12	14	16	18	20
3	6	9	12	15	18	21	24	27	30
4	8	12	16	20	24	28	32	36	40
5	10	15	20	25	30	35	40	45	50
6	12	18	24	30	36	42	48	54	60
7	14	21	28	35	42	49	56	63	70
8	16	24	32	40	48	56	64	72	80
9	18	27	36	45	54	63	72	81	90
10	20	30	40	50	60	70	80	90	100

To multiply 7×6 go along the 7 row and down the 6 column, where they meet gives the answer. Therefore $7 \times 6 = 42$

To divide 45 by 9. Find 9 on the top row and follow the column down until you reach 45, then follow the line across until you reach the left hand column, which gives the answer. Therefore $45 \div 9 = 5$

52. Place value

1	000	000	000	.	giga		G			10^9
	1	000	000	.	mega		M			10^6
		1	000	.	kilo		k			10^3
			100	.	hecto		h			10^2
			10	.	deca		da			10^1
			1				unit			1
d		deci	0	.	1					10^{-1}
c		centi	0	.	01					10^{-2}
m		milli	0	.	001					10^{-3}
μ		micro	0	.	000	001				10^{-6}
n		nano	0	.	000	000	001			10^{-9}
p		pico	0	.	000	000	000	001		10^{-12}

The above chart gives the number, the name, the abbreviation and the exponential form of the unit

53. Decimals: multiplication and division

To multiply by	Move the decimal point
10.00	1 place to the right
100.00	2 places to the right
1000.00	3 places to the right

Example

To multiply 5.432 by 10 000.
Move the decimal point 4 places to the right
= 54320.00

To divide by	Move the decimal point
10.00	1 place to the left
100.00	2 places to the left
1000.00	3 places to the left

Example

To divide 5.432 by 10 000.
Move the decimal point 4 places to the left
= 0.0005432

54. Circles

MEASUREMENTS

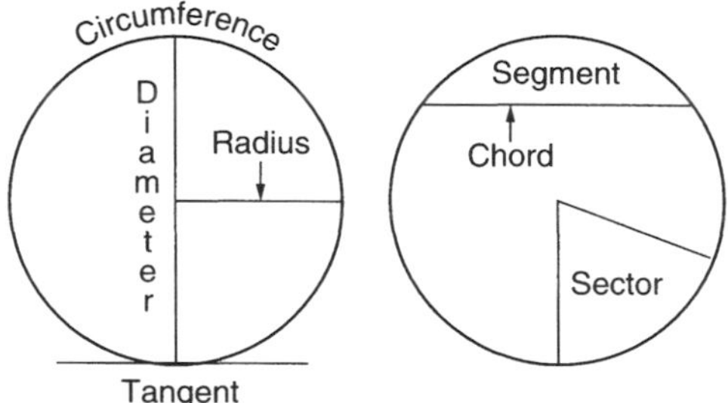

$$\text{Circumference} = \pi \times \text{diameter}$$
$$= \pi D$$
$$\text{or} = 2 \times \pi \times \text{radius}$$
$$= 2\pi r$$
$$\text{Area of a circle} = \pi \times \text{radius}^2$$
$$= \pi r^2$$

A circle has 360°

$$\pi = \text{pi} = \frac{22}{7}$$
$$= 3.142$$

$$1 \text{ Radian} = \frac{180^\circ}{\pi}$$
$$= 57.3^\circ$$

55. Similar triangles

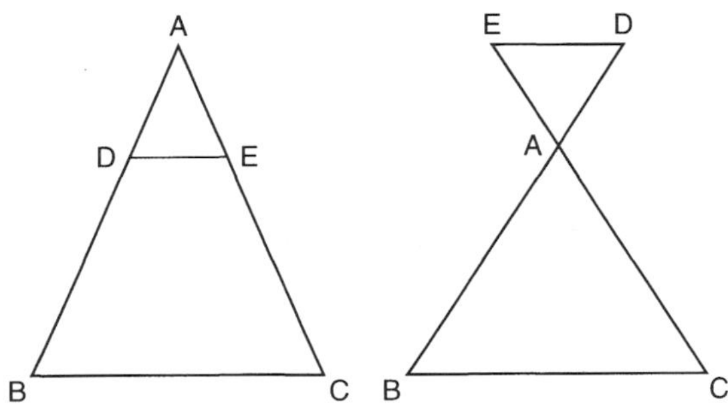

AD is proportional to AB
AE is proportional to AC
DE is proportional to BC

Angle ADE = Angle ABC
Angle EAD = Angle BAC
Angle DEA = Angle ACB

56. Triangles

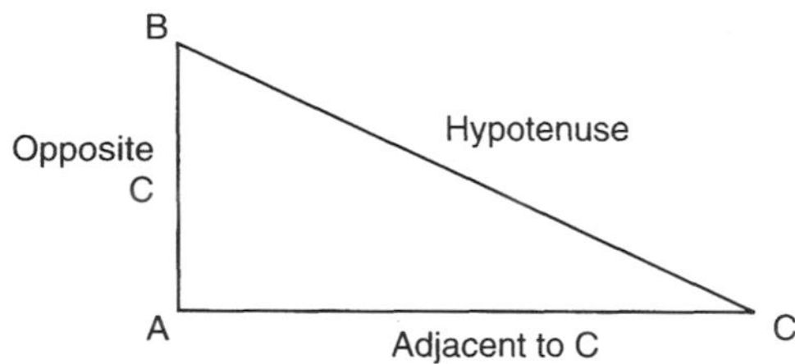

The three angles of all triangles add up to 180°
In the above, angle A = 90°
BC is opposite the right angle and is called the hypotenuse
AB is described as being opposite angle C
AC is described as being adjacent to angle C

PYTHAGORAS

$$AC^2 = AB^2 + BC^2$$

Example

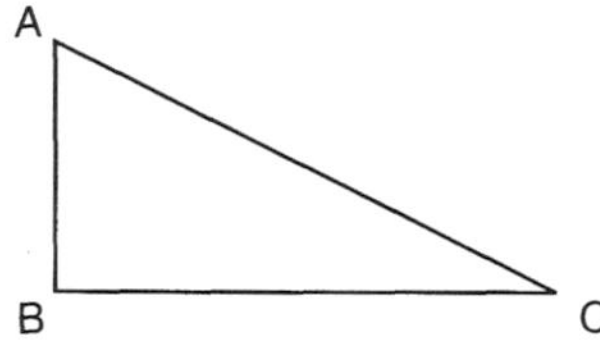

If AB = 5 cm and BC = 18.66 cm, find the length of AC

$$AC^2 = AB^2 + BC^2$$

$$AC^2 = 5^2 + 18.66^2$$

$$= 25 + 348.20$$

$$= 373.20$$

$$AC = \sqrt{373.20}$$

Therefore AC = 19.32 cm

IN ANY RIGHT-ANGLE TRIANGLE

$$\text{Tangent of an angle} = \frac{\text{opposite}}{\text{adjacent}}$$

$$\text{Sine of an angle} = \frac{\text{opposite}}{\text{hypotenuse}}$$

$$\text{Cosine of an angle} = \frac{\text{adjacent}}{\text{hypotenuse}}$$

Example

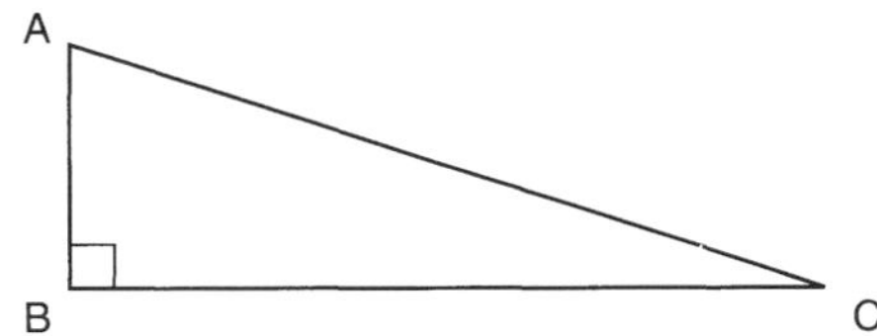

TANGENT

If angle ACB = 15° and AB = 5 cm, find BC

$$\text{tangent ACB} = \frac{AB}{BC}$$

$$BC = \frac{AB}{\tan ACB}$$

$$= \frac{5}{\tan 15^\circ}$$

On a calculator:

5	÷	15	tan	=	18.66

Therefore BC = 18.66 cm

SINE

If angle ACB = 15° and AB = 5 cm, find AC

$$\text{sine ACB} = \frac{AB}{AC}$$

$$AC = \frac{AB}{\sin ACB}$$

$$= \frac{5}{\sin 15^\circ}$$

On a calculator:

5	÷	15	sin	=	19.32

Therefore AC = 19.32 cm

COSINE

If angle ACB = 15° and BC = 18.66 cm, find AC

$$\text{cosine ACB} = \frac{BC}{AC}$$

$$AC = \frac{BC}{\cos ACB}$$

$$= \frac{18.66}{\cos 15^\circ}$$

On a calculator:

18.66	÷	15	cos	=	19.32

Therefore AC = 19.32 cm

57. Gradient

The gradient equals the slope of a line

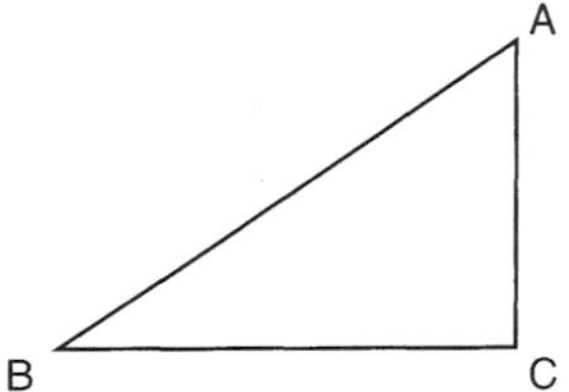

$$\text{To calculate the slope of AB} = \frac{\text{height}}{\text{distance}}$$

$$= \frac{\text{AC}}{\text{BC}}$$

Example

If AC = 6 and BC = 3, find the gradient

$$\text{AB} = \frac{6}{3}$$

Therefore the gradient of AB = 2

58. Vectors

Vectors are described as having direction and magnitude
Magnitude can be velocity, speed, weight, time, temperature, etc.
Vectors can be represented diagrammatically, by using triangles

EQUAL VECTORS

Vectors are said to be equal if they have the same magnitude and direction

INVERSE VECTORS

Vectors are said to be inverse if they have the same magnitude but are in opposite directions

TRIANGLE LAW

If you have two vectors (A and B), the result is equal to the length and direction of the line needed to complete the triangle (C)

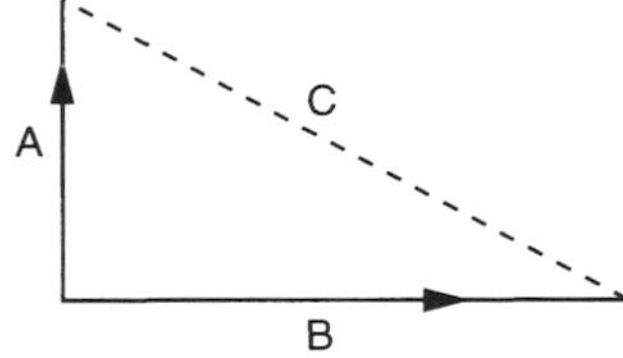

Example

If a person walks 5 km in an easterly direction and then 3 km in a northerly direction what is the shortest distance to return to the starting point?

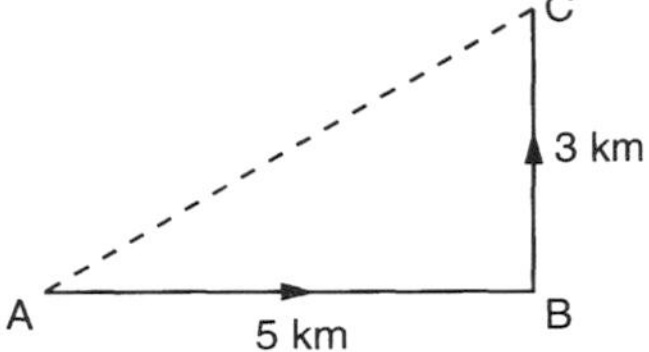

Using Pythagoras:

$$AB^2 + BC^2 = AC^2$$
$$5^2 + 3^2 = AC^2$$
$$25 + 9 = AC^2$$
$$AC = \sqrt{34}$$
$$= 5.8\,\text{km}$$

Therefore the shortest distance = 5.8 km

RECTANGLE OF VECTORS

Two vectors may be added to produce a rectangle of vectors. For example, if you have a force (N) acting at $y°$, find the horizontal (H) and vertical (V) components

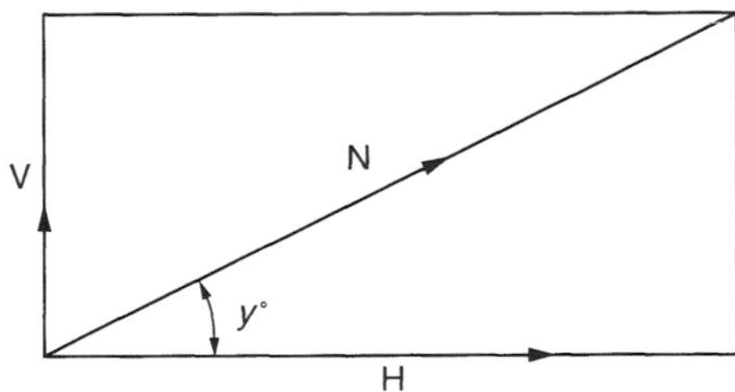

Example

A person's foot experiences a force of 6.8 kN at an angle to the ground of 60°. Resolve the resultant force into its vertical and horizontal components

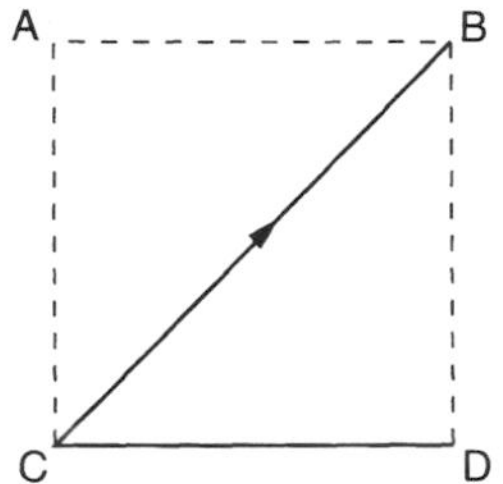

$$\angle BCD = 60^\circ$$

$$CB = 6.8\,\text{kN}$$

$$\text{Cos BCD} = \frac{\text{adjacent}}{\text{hypotenuse}} = \frac{CD}{CB}$$

$$\begin{aligned} CD &= \cos BCD \times CB \\ &= \cos 60^\circ \times 6.8 \\ &= 0.5 \times 6.8 \\ &= 3.4 \end{aligned}$$

Therefore the horizontal force = 3.4 kN

$$\sin BCD = \frac{\text{opposite}}{\text{hypotenuse}} = \frac{BD}{CB}$$

$$\begin{aligned} BD &= \sin BCD \times CB \\ &= \sin 60^\circ \times 6.8 \\ &= 0.866 \times 6.8 \\ &= 5.889 \end{aligned}$$

Therefore the vertical force = 5.89 kN

59. Indices

$y^2 = y \times y$

If y = 5:

$5^2 = 5 \times 5 = 25$

$y^3 = y \times y \times y$

If y = 5

$5^3 = 5 \times 5 \times 5 = 125$

On a calculator:

To find y^2 if y = 10

10	INV	x^2	=	100

To find y^3 if $y = 5$

5	x^y	3	=	125

To find y^4 if $y = 5$

5	x^y	4	=	625

60. Roots

A square root, symbol √, is the opposite of a^2. Therefore, if $a = 5$:

Example 1

$5^2 = 5 \times 5 = 25$

$\sqrt{25} = 5$

On a calculator:

25	√	=	5

Example 2

$5^3 = 5 \times 5 \times 5 = 125$

$3\sqrt{125} = 5$

On a calculator:

125	INV	$^3\sqrt{}$	=	5

Example 3

$5^4 = 5 \times 5 \times 5 \times 5 = 625$

$4\sqrt{625} = 5$

On a calculator:

625	INV	$x^{1/y}$	4	=	5

61. Fractions

TERMINOLOGY

$$\frac{\text{Numerator}}{\text{Denominator}}$$

Example

$$\frac{3}{4}$$

3 = the numerator
4 = the denominator

The lowest common multiple is the smallest number that all the denominators will divide into equally

Example

The lowest common multiple of 4 and 7 = 28

The lowest common multiple of 4 and 2 = 4

The lowest common multiple of 4 and 5 = 20

The lowest common multiple of 4 and 12 = 12

ADDING FRACTIONS

METHOD

1 Find the lowest common multiple

2 Change the fractions so that they all have the same denominator, i.e. divide the lowest common multiple by the original denominator

3 Multiply the numerator by the answer

4 Repeat for each fraction

5 Add the numerators

Example

$$\frac{3}{4}+\frac{2}{5}$$

The lowest common multiple of 4 and 5 = **20**

For the first fraction:

$20 \div 4 = 5$

$5 \times 3 = \mathbf{15}$

For the second fraction:

$20 \div 5 = 4$

$4 \times 2 = \mathbf{8}$

Therefore:

$$\frac{15}{20}+\frac{8}{20}=\frac{15+8}{20}=\frac{23}{20}$$

To find the whole number, divide the denominator into the numerator:

$$=1\frac{3}{20}$$

SUBTRACTING FRACTIONS

METHOD

1 Find the lowest common multiple

2 Change the fractions so that they all have the same denominator, i.e. divide the common multiple by the original denominator

3 Multiply the numerator by the answer

4 Repeat for each fraction

5 Subtract the numerators

Example

$$\frac{3}{4} - \frac{2}{5}$$

The lowest common multiple of 4 and 5 = **20**

For the first fraction:

$20 \div 4 = 5$

$5 \times 3 = \mathbf{15}$

For the second fraction:

$20 \div 5 = 4$

$4 \times 2 = \mathbf{8}$

Therefore:

$$\frac{15}{20} - \frac{8}{20}$$

$$= \frac{15 - 8}{20} = \frac{7}{20}$$

FRACTIONS: MULTIPLYING AND DIVIDING

MULTIPLYING FRACTIONS

1 Multiply the numerators together

2 Multiply the denominators together

Example

$$\frac{3}{4} \times \frac{2}{5} = \frac{6}{20}$$

Reducing the fraction to the lowest terms (in this example by dividing the top and bottom by 2), which gives:

$$\frac{3}{10}$$

DIVIDING FRACTIONS

1 Turn the second fraction upside down

2 Multiply

Example

$$\begin{aligned} &\frac{3}{4} \div \frac{2}{5} \\ &= \frac{3}{4} \times \frac{5}{2} \\ &= \frac{15}{8} \\ &= 1\frac{7}{8} \end{aligned}$$

62. Percentage

Percentage = parts per 100
Symbol = %

TO CHANGE A DECIMAL TO A PERCENTAGE

Multiply by 100

Example

$$0.45 \times 100 = 45\%$$

TO CHANGE A FRACTION TO A PERCENTAGE

Multiply by 100

Example

$$\frac{2}{7} \times \frac{100}{1} = \frac{200}{7} = 28.57\%$$

TO FIND A PERCENTAGE OF A QUANTITY

1 Divide the percentage by 100

2 Multiply the answer by the number you are finding the % of

Example

15% of 130

$$\frac{15}{100} \times 130 = 19.5\%$$

63. Ratio

Ratio is another word for parts, e.g. if a drug is diluted in a solution at a ratio of 50 mg/ml, there would be:

- 50 mg of the drug
- 1 ml of solution

NB:

- 1 in 4 means 1 part of a solution in 4 parts of a diluted solution, giving a total of 4 parts
- 1:3 means 1 part of a solution added to 3 parts of diluted solution, giving a total of 4 parts

Example 1

Change 1 in 6 to a ratio

$6 - 1 = 5$ parts of diluted solution

Therefore the ratio is 1:5

Example 2

Change 1:7 to 1 in ?

1:7 = 8 parts

Therefore = 1 in 8

64. Equations: equals signs

MOVEMENT ACROSS AN EQUALS SIGN

Plus become minus
Minus becomes plus
Multiplication becomes division
Division becomes multiplication

EXAMPLE

$$6 = 3y - 9$$
$$6 + 9 = 3y$$
$$15 = 3y$$
$$\frac{15}{3} = y$$
$$5 = y$$

CROSS MULTIPLICATION

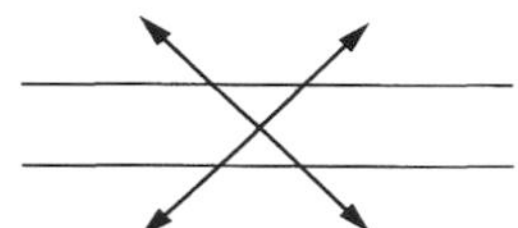

Movement is in either direction across an = sign
All parts of the equation must be included
There is no change of sign

Example 1

$$\frac{2y}{4} = \frac{3}{5}$$

$$y = \frac{4 \times 3}{2 \times 5}$$

$$= \frac{12}{10}$$

Example 2

$$\frac{2y}{4} = \frac{3}{5} + \frac{6}{7}$$

$$y = \frac{4 \times 3}{2 \times 5} + \frac{4 \times 6}{2 \times 7}$$

$$= \frac{12}{10} + \frac{24}{14}$$

$$y = 2\frac{32}{35}$$

65. Simultaneous equations

METHOD

1 Express x in terms of y in one equation

2 Substitute the answer found for x in another equation so that the whole of the equation is in terms of y

3 Calculate y

4 Substitute the answer for y in an equation

5 Calculate x

Example 1

1) $3x + 2y = 12$
2) $x + 5y = 17$

Taking equation 2, write it in terms of y:

$$x + 5y = 17$$
$$x = 17 - 5y$$

Substituting in equation 1:

$$3x + 2y = 12$$
$$3(17 - 5y) + 2y = 12$$
$$51 - 15y + 2y = 12$$
$$51 - 12 = 13y$$
$$39 = 13y$$
$$\frac{39}{13} = y$$
$$y = 3$$

Substituting for y in equation 2:

$$x + 5y = 17$$
$$x + 5 \times 3 = 17$$
$$x = 17 - 15$$
$$x = 2$$

Therefore $x = 2$ and $y = 3$

Example 2

1) $3x + 2y = 12$
2) $4x + 5y = 23$

Taking equation 1, write in terms of y:

$$3x + 2y = 12$$
$$3x = 12 - 2y$$
$$x = \frac{12}{3} - \frac{2y}{3}$$

Substituting in equation 2:

$$4x + 5y = 23$$
$$4(\frac{12}{3} - \frac{2y}{3}) + 5y = 23$$
$$16 - \frac{8y}{3} + 5y = 23$$
$$\frac{-8y}{3} + \frac{15y}{3} = 23 - 16$$
$$\frac{7y}{3} = 7$$
$$7y = 21$$
$$y = 3$$

Substituting for y in equation 1:

$$3x + 2y = 12$$
$$3x + 2 \times 3 = 12$$
$$3x = 12 - 6$$
$$3x = 6$$
$$x = 2$$

Therefore $y = 3$ and $x = 2$

66. Logarithms

Logarithms are used to enable large numbers to be handled easily. Following the introduction of calculators they are now mainly used to enable large ranges of numbers to be portrayed graphically and in the simplification of complex formulae

Although logarithms can be to any base, in practice they are usually to base 10 or to base e (e = exponential number = 2.718)

DEFINITION

The logarithm is the power by which the base must be raised to give the number

Example

10 = 10^1 therefore logarithm = 1
100 = 10^2 therefore logarithm = 2
1000 = 10^3 therefore logarithm = 3
10 000 = 10^4 therefore logarithm = 4

NB: To multiply log numbers, add them together

On a calculator:

To find the logarithm of a number:

Enter the number **log**

To find the log of 1.234

1.234 log = 0.0913

67. Calculus

DIFFERENTIATION

Formula

$$\frac{d(x^n)}{dx} = (n)x^{n-1}$$

To differentiate:

1 Multiply by the index n

2 Reduce the index by 1

Example

x^3 becomes $3x^2$
x^5 becomes $5x^4$

INTEGRATION

Formula

$$\int x^n.dx = \frac{x^{n+1}}{(n+1)}$$

To integrate:

1 Add 1 to the index

2 Divide by the index plus 1

3 Substitute x with the top integer

4 Substitute x with the bottom integer

5 Subtract the second equation from the first

Example

$$y = \int_{2}^{5} x^3 \cdot dx = \left[\frac{x^4}{4}\right]_2^5$$

$$y = \frac{5^4}{4} - \frac{2^4}{4}$$

$$y = \frac{(5 \times 5 \times 5 \times 5)}{4} - \frac{(2 \times 2 \times 2 \times 2)}{4}$$

$$= \frac{625}{4} - \frac{16}{4}$$

$$= 156.25 - 4$$

$$= 152.25$$

Therefore $y = 152.25$

68. Calculator glossary

Constant factor enter the number and press either +, −, ×, or ÷ twice to add, subtract, multiply or divide by the same number for a number of calculations

Cosine enter the number and press cos

Cosine^{-1} enter the number and press INV and $\cos^{-1}$

Cube a number enter the number and press x^y, 3 and =

Logarithms enter the number and press log

Memory use Min after the first calculation, M+ after each following calculation and MR to find the total

Negative numbers enter the number and press +/−

Pi press either EXP or π

Radian 57.3 degrees

Root enter the number you wish to find the root of and press INV, $X^{1/y}$, the root number and =

Sine enter the number and press sin

Sine^{-1} enter the number and press INV and $\sin^{-1}$

Square a number enter the number and press INV and x^2

Square root enter the number and press $\sqrt{}$

Tangent enter the number and press tan

Tangent^{-1} enter the number and press INV and $\tan^{-1}$

Further reading

Ball J, Price A 1995 Chesney's radiographic imaging. Blackwell Science, Oxford

Bradbeer R, Bawtree M 1979 The Sinclair book of students' calculations. Martin Books, in association with Sinclair Radionics Ltd (Huntingdon), Cambridge

Clegg F 1990 Simple statistics. Cambridge University Press, Cambridge

Dobinson J 1978 Mathematics for technology. Penguin Books, Middlesex

Gatford J D, Anderson R E 1998 Nursing calculations, 5th edn. Churchill Livingstone, Edinburgh

Graham D T 1996 Principles of radiological physics. Churchill Livingstone, New York

Greer A 1986 A complete GCSE mathematics. Stanley Thornes (Publishers) Ltd, Cheltenham

Gunn C 1994 Radiographic imaging. Churchill Livingstone, Edinburgh

Hall S 1991 Basic biomechanics. Mosby Year Book, St Louis

Miller S 1991 Experimental Design and Statistics. Routledge, London

Neave HR 2000 Elementary statistics tables. Routledge, London

Ozkaya N 1991 Fundamentals of biomechanics. Van Nostrand Reinhold